Department of Veterans Affairs
Health Services Research & Development Service | Evidence-based Synthesis Program

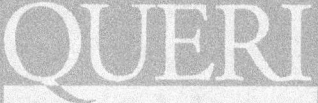

Predictors and Consequences of Severe Hypoglycemia in Adults with Diabetes – A Systematic Review of the Evidence

April 2012

Prepared for:
Department of Veterans Affairs
Veterans Health Administration
Quality Enhancement Research Initiative
Health Services Research & Development Service
Washington, DC 20420

Prepared by:
Evidence-based Synthesis Program (ESP) Center
Minneapolis VA Medical Center
Minneapolis, MN
Timothy J. Wilt, M.D., M.P.H., Director

Investigators:
Principal Investigator:
Hanna E. Bloomfield, M.D., M.P.H.

Co-Investigators:
Nancy Greer, Ph.D.
David Newman, M.D.

Research Associates:
Roderick MacDonald, M.S.
Maureen Carlyle, M.P.H.
Patrick Fitzgerald, M.P.H.
Indulis Rutks, B.S.

This report is for internal use of the Department of Veterans Affairs and should not be distributed outside the agency.

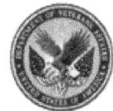
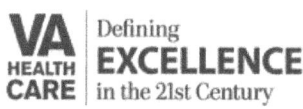

PREFACE

Quality Enhancement Research Initiative's (QUERI) Evidence-based Synthesis Program (ESP) was established to provide timely and accurate syntheses of targeted healthcare topics of particular importance to Veterans Affairs (VA) managers and policymakers, as they work to improve the health and healthcare of Veterans. The ESP disseminates these reports throughout VA.

QUERI provides funding for four ESP Centers and each Center has an active VA affiliation. The ESP Centers generate evidence syntheses on important clinical practice topics, and these reports help:

- develop clinical policies informed by evidence,
- guide the implementation of effective services to improve patient outcomes and to support VA clinical practice guidelines and performance measures, and
- set the direction for future research to address gaps in clinical knowledge.

In 2009, the ESP Coordinating Center was created to expand the capacity of QUERI Central Office and the four ESP sites by developing and maintaining program processes. In addition, the Center established a Steering Committee comprised of QUERI field-based investigators, VA Patient Care Services, Office of Quality and Performance, and Veterans Integrated Service Networks (VISN) Clinical Management Officers. The Steering Committee provides program oversight, guides strategic planning, coordinates dissemination activities, and develops collaborations with VA leadership to identify new ESP topics of importance to Veterans and the VA healthcare system.

Comments on this evidence report are welcome and can be sent to Nicole Floyd, ESP Coordinating Center Program Manager, at nicole.floyd@va.gov.

Recommended citation: Bloomfield HE, Greer N, Newman D, MacDonald R, Carlyle M, Fitzgerald P, Rutks I, and Wilt, TJ. Predictors and Consequences of Severe Hypoglycemia in Adults with Diabetes – A Systematic Review of the Evidence. VA-ESP Project #09-009; 2012.

This report is based on research conducted by the Evidence-based Synthesis Program (ESP) Center located at the Minneapolis VA Medical Center, Minneapolis, MN funded by the Department of Veterans Affairs, Veterans Health Administration, Office of Research and Development, Quality Enhancement Research Initiative. The findings and conclusions in this document are those of the author(s) who are responsible for its contents; the findings and conclusions do not necessarily represent the views of the Department of Veterans Affairs or the United States government. Therefore, no statement in this article should be construed as an official position of the Department of Veterans Affairs. No investigators have any affiliations or financial involvement (e.g., employment, consultancies, honoraria, stock ownership or options, expert testimony, grants or patents received or pending, or royalties) that conflict with material presented in the report.

TABLE OF CONTENTS

FIGURES

APPENDIX A. SEARCH STRATEGIES

EXECUTIVE SUMMARY

BACKGROUND

Prevalence of type 2 diabetes is increasing at an alarming pace, fueled by the rising rates of overweight and obesity in many populations. In the VA healthcare system, the prevalence of diabetes was 20% in fiscal year 2000 and is now estimated at nearly 25%.

Although people with diabetes have a substantially increased risk of cardiovascular disease (CVD), recent trials show that intensive glucose lowering does not reduce the risk of CVD death or all-cause mortality although it reduces the risk of microvascular complications (nephropathy, retinopathy and neuropathy) and possibly non-fatal myocardial infarction. Intensive glucose control also increases the risk of hypoglycemic episodes. Several recent meta-analyses of the trials comparing intensive to conventional glucose control concluded that intensive control is associated with a 2-2.5 fold increased risk of severe hypoglycemia. The reviews however have not included smaller randomized trials, trials focused on the comparison of specific drug regimens, and non-randomized trials. We conducted the current review to provide broader insight into the incidence of, the risk factors for, and the clinical and social impact of severe hypoglycemia in adults with type 2 diabetes treated with glucose lowering medications.

The key questions were as follows: In adults with type 2 diabetes treated with one or more hypoglycemic agents:

Key Question #1: What is the **incidence** of severe hypoglycemia in adults with type 2 diabetes on one or more hypoglycemic agents?

Key Question #2: What are the **risk factors** for severe hypoglycemia in adults with type 2 diabetes on one or more hypoglycemic agents (e.g., demographics, co-morbidities, diabetes treatment regimen, other medication use, goal and achieved HbA1c)?

Key Question #3: What is the effect of severe hypoglycemia on other **outcomes** in adults with type 2 diabetes on one or more hypoglycemic agents (e.g., quality of life, mortality, morbidity, utilization)?

METHODS

We searched MEDLINE (OVID) for clinical trials and systematic reviews from 1950 to through November 2011 using standard search terms. Studies were eligible if they involved adults with type 2 diabetes, were published in the English language and reported outcomes of interest. Search terms included: hypoglycemia, hypoglycaemia, and diabetes mellitus, type 2. The search was not limited to randomized controlled trials (RCTs). We obtained additional articles from a search of the Cochrane Library, other systematic reviews, reference lists of pertinent studies, reviews, editorials and expert consultation. We defined severe hypoglycemia as an episode with typical symptoms resolving after treatment administered by another person.

Investigators and research assistants trained in the critical analysis of literature assessed for relevance the abstracts of citations identified from literature searches. Full-text articles of potentially relevant abstracts were retrieved for further review. For Key Questions #1 and #2, we excluded studies with fewer than 500 patients or duration less than 6 months. We also excluded studies if the medications involved were not FDA approved. For Key Question #3, there were no restrictions on sample size or study duration.

Study characteristics, patient characteristics, and outcomes were extracted by investigators and trained research associates under the supervision of the Principal Investigator. We assessed study quality according to established criteria for randomized trials and non-randomized trials.

DATA SYNTHESIS

We constructed evidence tables showing the study characteristics for all included studies. Outcomes tables were organized by key question. We critically analyzed studies to compare their characteristics, methods, and findings. We compiled a summary of findings for each key question or clinical topic, and drew conclusions based on qualitative synthesis of the findings or pooled results, where appropriate. We identified and highlighted findings from veteran populations.

PEER REVIEW

A draft version of this report was reviewed by technical experts, as well as clinical leadership. Reviewer comments were addressed and our responses may be found in Appendix C.

RESULTS

We reviewed 2353 titles and abstracts from the electronic search. After applying inclusion/exclusion criteria at the abstract level, 1914 references were excluded. We retrieved 439 full-text articles for further review and another 320 references were excluded. We identified 8 references by hand searching reference lists of relevant publications resulting in a total of 127 references for inclusion in the current review.

Key Question #1. What is the incidence of severe hypoglycemia in adults with type 2 diabetes on one or more hypoglycemic agents?

Overall incidence of severe hypoglycemia was less than 1% in most of the 60 reviewed studies, particularly those of metformin monotherapy (<1%), glucagon-like peptide-1 (GLP-1) analogs (< 1%), dipeptidyl-peptidase-4 (DPP-4) inhibitors (<1%), insulin detemir (<1%), glinides (0%) and thiazolidinediones (TZDs) (<1%). Annual rates of severe hypoglycemia were greater than 1% for sulfonylureas and the following insulin preparations: neutral protamine Hagedorn (NPH), glargine, lispro and glulisine. Some of the highest rates of severe hypoglycemia were seen in trials of intensive glucose control.

We reviewed an additional 16 studies to gain a broader population-based perspective on incidence of symptomatic hypoglycemia (defined more broadly than "severe"): 13 were survey studies reporting patient-recalled rates. Eleven of these 13 asked patients to report on events in the past 6 months (N=6) to one year (N=5). In these 11 studies, patient reported incidences of symptomatic hypoglycemia varied widely from 1% to 17%, likely due to a wide range of study designs, populations, and lengths of follow-up.

Limitations

Much of the evidence comes from reports of RCTs funded by pharmaceutical companies which enroll highly selected populations and generally do not include those at highest risk for hypoglycemia. Furthermore, the definitions of severe hypoglycemia varied among studies and there is likely substantial ascertainment bias, especially in the RCTs designed primarily to measure the benefits of specific drug regimens.

Discussion

The incidence of severe hypoglycemia ranges from 0-3% per year for adults with type 2 diabetes on hypoglycemic medications. Incidence is highest in studies of people on insulins, sulfonylureas and regimens targeting intensive control of hemoglobin A1c (HbA1c) levels. Risk is negligible for people on metformin, GLP-1 analogs, DPP-4 inhibitors, glinides and TZDs. The incidence was more than 2-fold greater among patients undergoing intensive control compared with conventional control. The most important limitation of the data is that they were mostly derived from industry funded randomized trials of highly selected populations. A review of survey data from more representative populations suggests that the incidence of symptomatic hypoglycemia may be more common than reported in these trials.

Key Question #2. What are the risk factors for severe hypoglycemia in adults with type 2 diabetes on one or more hypoglycemic agents (e.g., demographics, co-morbidities, diabetes treatment regimen, other medication use, goal and achieved HbA1c)?

We identified 14 articles from 12 studies that reported multivariate adjusted risk factor analyses for severe hypoglycemia in adults with type 2 diabetes on hypoglycemic mediations. Since these varied considerably with respect to risk factors evaluated (and their definitions), populations studied, and lengths of follow-up, the data were considered unsuitable for pooling. Transient causes (e.g., missed meal, excess exercise, alcohol use, acute infection) were not included.

Independent risk factors for severe hypoglycemia in persons with type 2 diabetes on hypoglycemic medication include: intensive glycemic control, history of hypoglycemia, renal insufficiency, history of microvascular complications, longer diabetes duration, lower education level, African American race and history of dementia. Gender, age and BMI are not consistently associated with risk, although in the two largest studies, higher age and lower BMI were significantly associated with higher risk.

Limitations

We were unable to pool results across studies due to the heterogeneity of the study designs, analytical methods and risk factors assessed. Furthermore, the data are relatively sparse and almost certainly reflect publication bias.

Discussion

The literature in this area is relatively sparse. We did not identify any other systematic reviews that evaluated risk factors for severe hypoglycemia in people with type 2 diabetes, although our findings are generally consistent with what has been summarized elsewhere. The most important limitation of the data is that there is likely publication bias since negative analyses are less likely to be published. In addition several potential risk factors (e.g., recent hospital discharge, smoking status, polypharmacy, alcohol consumption) have not been adequately evaluated.

Key Question #3. What is the effect of severe hypoglycemia on other outcomes in adults with type 2 diabetes on one or more hypoglycemic agents (e.g., quality of life, mortality, morbidity, utilization)?

We identified 53 studies (in 59 articles) that provided outcomes data from patients who experienced severe hypoglycemia. Overall, we found good evidence for an increased risk of the following outcomes: all-cause mortality, neurological events (other than non-fatal stroke), hospital and emergency department utilization and decreased quality of life. We found limited data about non-fatal MI, non-fatal stroke, cognitive decline, motor vehicle accidents, falls and traumatic injuries, work productivity and other medical service utilization.

Limitations

Few studies that address outcomes of severe hypoglycemic episodes include appropriate control groups. In addition, many outcomes of interest were not widely reported.

Discussion

Episodes of severe hypoglycemia may be a marker of serious illness and observed clinical outcomes may be due to illness rather than severe hypoglycemia. Similarly, it is unclear whether severe hypoglycemia contributes to cognitive decline or whether individuals experience more episodes of severe hypoglycemia as a result of cognitive decline.

FUTURE RESEARCH RECOMMENDATIONS

Key Question #1 and Key Question #2: Larger population-based prospective studies of people on a variety of hypoglycemic agents that employ accurate methods for ascertaining incidence of severe hypoglycemia should be performed. Studies should control for or stratify outcomes by important patient, disease and comorbidity factors including: age, gender, race/ethnicity, socio-economic and marital status, disease duration and severity (e.g., HbA1c level, presence or absence of diabetic complications).

Key Question #3: Future studies of outcomes associated with severe hypoglycemia should be prospective, use a uniform and generally accepted definition of severe hypoglycemia and include as controls people with medication-treated diabetes who have not experienced severe hypoglycemia. Also, studies should clearly distinguish between short-term or episode-related versus long-term consequences.

EVIDENCE REPORT

INTRODUCTION

Prevalence of type 2 diabetes is increasing at an alarming pace, fueled by the rising rates of overweight and obesity in many populations. A recent study estimated that the number of people with diabetes increased worldwide from 153 million in 1980 to 347 million in 2008.[1] This study estimated that from 1980 to 2008, the age standardized prevalence of diabetes in the United States increased from 6% to 12% in men and from 5% to 9% in women. In the VA, prevalence of diabetes is higher than in the general population and increasing over time. Miller et al. reported estimated rates of diabetes in VA of 17% in fiscal year (FY) 1998, 19% in FY99 and 20% in FY00.[2] More recently, it was estimated that nearly 25% of veterans receiving care in the VA have diabetes (http://www.va.gov/health/NewsFeatures/20110321a.asp, accessed April 3, 2012).

Although people with diabetes have a substantially increased risk of cardiovascular disease (CVD), three large well designed recent clinical trials testing intensive versus conventional glucose control strategies (ACCORD[3], ADVANCE[4] and VA-DT[5]), have found that intensive glucose control does not reduce the risk of CVD death or all-cause mortality although it reduces the risk of microvascular complications (nephropathy, retinopathy and neuropathy)[6] and possibly non-fatal myocardial infarction.[7] Intensive glucose control also increases the risk of hypoglycemic episodes. Several recent meta-analyses that included these large "intensive versus conventional control" trials have concluded that intensive control is associated with a 2-2.5 fold increased risk of severe hypoglycemia.[8-11] However, these reviews included only randomized controlled trials; we are unaware of a comprehensive systematic review examining incidence of and risk factors for severe hypoglycemia in adults with type 2 diabetes in both real-world and clinical trial settings.

Despite the increased risk of hypoglycemia with intensive glycemic control, influential national guidelines support an aggressive approach for patients with type 2 diabetes, recommending a target hemoglobin A1c level (HbA1c) of less than 7.[12] This recommendation implies that the benefits of tight control outweigh the risks even though the balance between these benefits and harms is not actually known. In particular, the effects of hypoglycemia on outcomes besides CVD events and all-cause mortality have not, to our knowledge, been rigorously evaluated. The VA/DoD guidelines recommend a more nuanced approach: target HbA1c levels are based on life expectancy and severity of microvascular complications. A level of < 7% is recommended only for those with no microvascular complications and a life expectancy of >10 years (http://www. healthquality.va.gov/diabetes_mellitus.asp, accessed January 27, 2012).

We conducted the current review to provide broader insight into the incidence of, the risk factors for, and the clinical impact of severe hypoglycemia in adults with type 2 diabetes treated with glucose lowering medications.

METHODS

TOPIC DEVELOPMENT

This project was nominated by Leonard Pogach, MD, National Program Director for Diabetes. The scope of the report and key questions were refined with input from a technical expert panel.

The key questions, as shown in the analytic framework in Figure 1, were as follows:

Key Question #1: What is the **incidence** of severe hypoglycemia in adults with type 2 diabetes on one or more hypoglycemic agents?

Key Question #2: What are the **risk factors** for severe hypoglycemia in adults with type 2 diabetes on one or more hypoglycemic agents (e.g., demographics, co-morbidities, diabetes treatment regimen, other medication use, goal and achieved HbA1c)?

Key Question #3: What is the effect of severe hypoglycemia on other **outcomes** in adults with type 2 diabetes on one or more hypoglycemic agents (e.g., quality of life, mortality, morbidity, utilization)?

Extension of Key Question #1: In order to gain a more population-based perspective on hypoglycemia incidence (as recommended by our technical expert panel November 1, 2011) we re-reviewed all the abstracts identified through the initial search strategy (through November, 2011) to find articles that might contain data from more representative groups that had not met the initial inclusion criteria.

SEARCH STRATEGY

We searched MEDLINE (OVID) for clinical trials and systematic reviews from 1950 to December 2010 using standard search terms. The search was updated in November 2011. We limited the search to articles involving adult, human subjects and published in the English language. Search terms included: hypoglycemia, hypoglycaemia, and diabetes mellitus, type 2. The full MEDLINE search strategy is presented in Appendix A.

We obtained additional articles from a search of the Cochrane Library, other systematic reviews, reference lists of pertinent studies, reviews, editorials, and by consulting experts. We also searched the following Web sites: Centers for Disease Control, ClinicalTrials.gov, Department of Transportation, Framingham Heart Study, National Health and Nutrition Examination Survey, National Institute of Diabetes and Digestive and Kidney Diseases, and Occupational Safety and Health Administration.

Figure 1. Analytic Framework

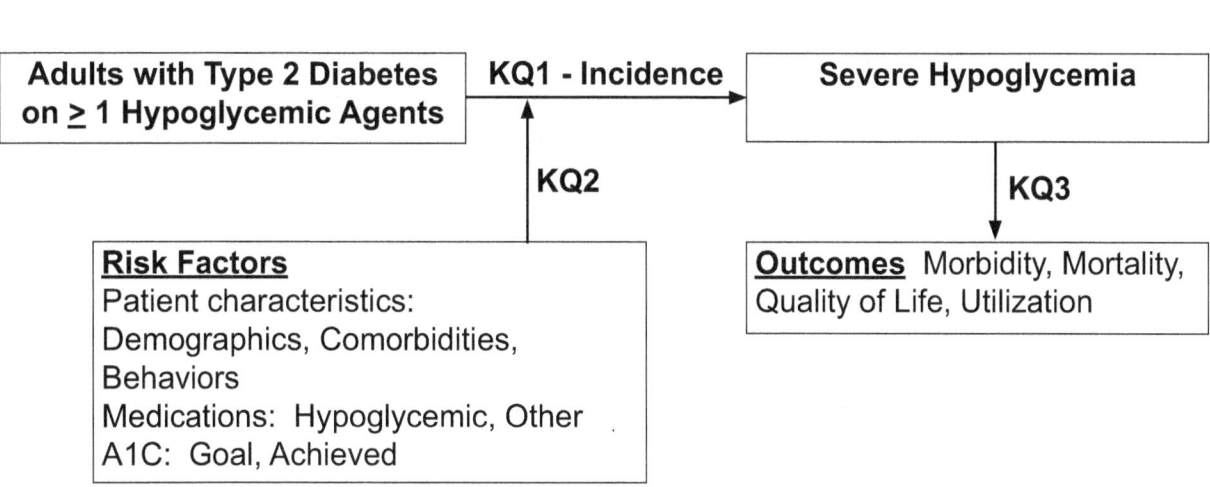

STUDY SELECTION

Investigators and research assistants trained in the critical analysis of literature assessed for relevance the abstracts of citations identified from literature searches. Full-text articles of potentially relevant abstracts were retrieved for further review.

Specific exclusion criteria for Key Questions #1 and #2 were as follows:

1. Population: exclude if animal study, age less than 18 years, inpatients, type 1 diabetes, patient on dialysis, gestational diabetes, or fasting populations.

2. Publication type: exclude case reports, narrative reviews, case series, letters, editorials, commentaries, book chapters, dissertations, other summaries, duplicate publications.

3. Outcomes: exclude if no outcomes of interest. Outcomes of interest are incidence of severe hypoglycemia and risk factors for severe hypoglycemia. Exclude if severe hypoglycemia not reported or defined.

4. Study duration: exclude if study is less than 6 months in duration.

5. Sample size: exclude if study enrolled fewer than 500 patients.

6. Intervention: exclude if study only includes patients on one or more non-FDA approved hypoglycemic agent (vildagliptin, algogliptin, taspoglutide, giclazide, troglitazone, exubera, any inhaled insulin) or on continuous insulin infusion.

For Key Question #1 – Extension, we employed the same exclusion criteria with the following modifications: we included population or clinic-based studies that may have enrolled fewer than 500 patients or had fewer than 6 months of follow-up; in which the definition of severe hypoglycemia may not have been rigorously defined but included some definition of symptomatic hypoglycemia; and in which there may not have been true incidence data (e.g., cross-sectional patient surveys). From this search we identified 16 articles (see Figure 2, shaded boxes).

For Key Question #3, we placed no restriction on sample size or study duration. The study had to report an association between severe hypoglycemia and outcomes of interest. Outcomes of interest included all-cause mortality, non-fatal myocardial infarction, non-fatal stroke, neurological events (other than stroke), hospitalizations, emergency department visits, accidents/ trauma, quality of life, cognitive function, productivity, and other health resource utilization.

DATA ABSTRACTION

We abstracted the following data for each included study (as appropriate based on study design): study design, definition of severe hypoglycemia, length of follow-up, population characteristics, subject inclusion and exclusion criteria, intervention(s), comparison(s), length of follow-up, and outcome(s).

QUALITY ASSESSMENT

We assessed study quality for randomized controlled trials using the criteria recommended by the Cochrane Collaboration to assess the risk of bias of studies included in a systematic review:[13] 1) adequate allocation concealment, based on the approach by Schulz and Grimes;[14] 2) blinding methods (participant, investigator, or outcome assessor); 3) how incomplete data were addressed (did the study analyze the data based on the intention-to-treat principle, i.e., were all subjects who were randomized included in the outcomes analyses), 4) reasons for dropouts/attrition reported. Studies were rated good, fair or of poor quality. A rating of good generally indicated that the trial reported adequate allocation concealment, blinding, analysis by intent-to-treat, and reasons for dropouts/attrition were reported. Studies were generally rated poor if the method of allocation concealment was inadequate, blinding was not defined, analysis by intent-to-treat was not utilized and reasons for dropouts/attrition were not reported and/or there was a high rate of attrition.

Quality assessment for non-randomized studies was based on: 1) population, 2) outcomes, 3) measurement, 4) confounding, and 5) intervention (if applicable). We assessed whether the study fulfilled the descriptive characteristics for each element (see Appendix B). Studies were considered to be of higher quality and more applicable if they were prospective, explicitly defined severe hypoglycemia, used multivariate analysis and included patients representative of typical patients with type 2 diabetes.

DATA SYNTHESIS

We constructed evidence tables showing the study characteristics for all included studies. Outcomes tables were organized by key question. We critically analyzed studies to compare their characteristics, methods, and findings. We compiled a summary of findings for each key question and drew conclusions based on qualitative synthesis of the findings or pooled results, where appropriate.

For Key Question #1, data were pooled and analyzed in Comprehensive Meta-Analysis software© (Biostat, Inc., Englewood, NJ). Risk ratios (RR) were calculated using a random-effects model if substantial heterogeneity was present. Statistical heterogeneity between trials was assessed using the I^2 test with a score of 50% or greater suggesting moderate to substantial heterogeneity among studies.

PEER REVIEW

A draft version of this report was reviewed by technical experts as well as clinical leadership. Their comments and our responses are shown in Appendix C.

RESULTS

LITERATURE FLOW

We reviewed 2353 titles and abstracts from the electronic search. After applying inclusion/ exclusion criteria at the abstract level, 1914 references were excluded. We retrieved 439 full-text articles for further review and another 320 references were excluded. We identified 8 references by hand searching reference lists of relevant publications resulting in a total of 127 references for inclusion in the current review. We grouped the studies by key question. We re-reviewed excluded studies to identify studies that might address a more population-based perspective on hypoglycemia incidence (Key Question #1-Extension). Sixteen articles were included in this extended view of incidence. Figure 2 details the exclusion criteria and the number of references related to each of the key questions.

Figure 2. Literature Flow Diagram

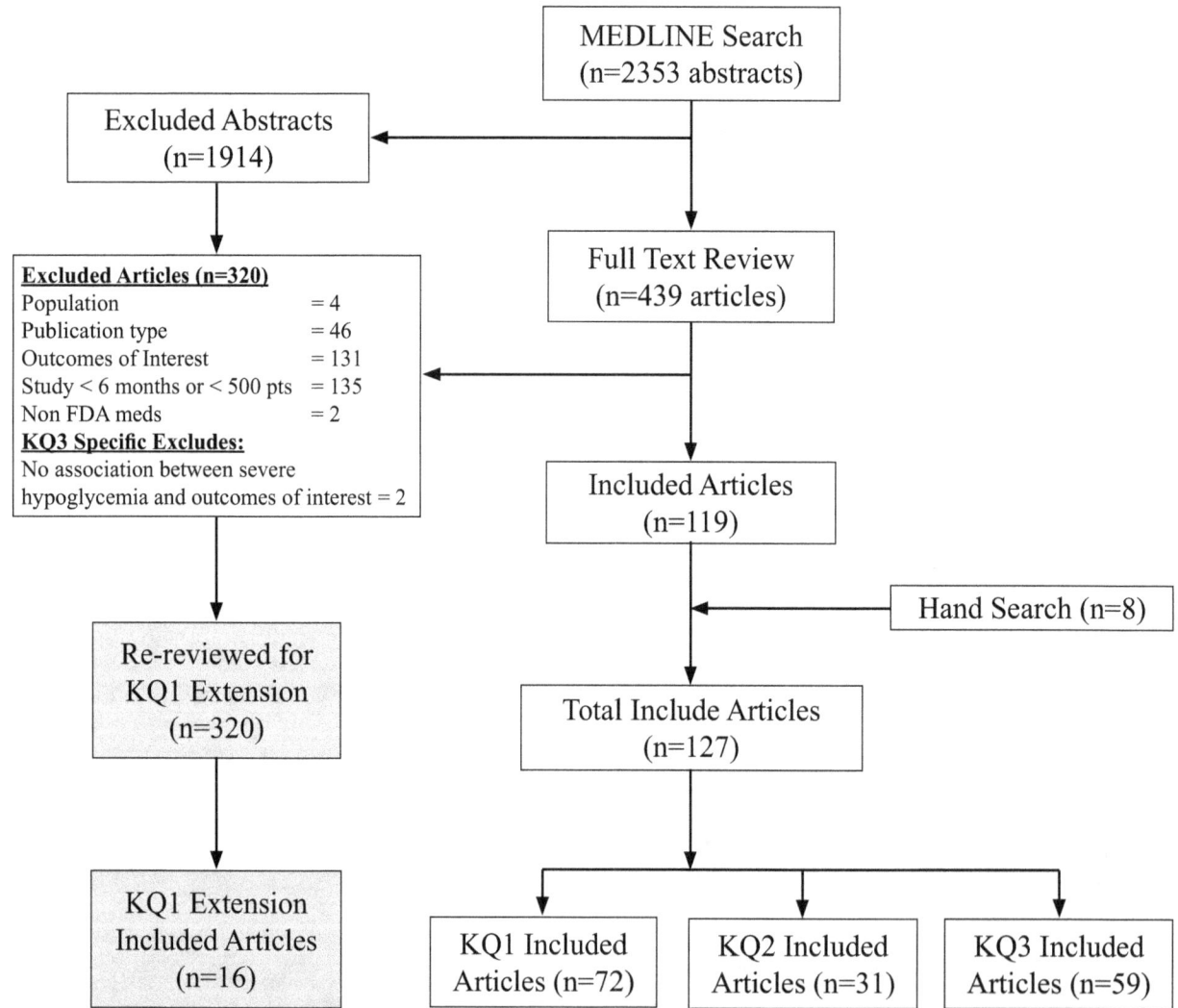

*A number of articles provided data for more than one KQ. Therefore, the total number of included articles does not equal the sum of the articles for each key question.

KEY QUESTION #1. What is the incidence of severe hypoglycemia in adults with type 2 diabetes on one or more hypoglycemic agents?

We identified 72 articles on 60 studies that provided data to address Key Question #1. We also identified 21 systematic reviews that were not funded by industry and provided severe hypoglycemia data. Four of the reviews included only the "intensive versus conventional" studies while 17 reviewed specific drugs or drug combinations.

Overview of Included Studies (Appendix E, Table 1)

The 60 studies included 46 RCTs (N>75,000), eight prospective observational studies,[15-22] and six retrospective studies.[23-28] Five of the RCTs randomized participants to an intensive versus a conventional treatment strategy, and not to specific drug regimens.[3-5, 21, 29, 30] Thirty were multinational, eighteen were conducted in the US and/or Canada, six in the United Kingdom, five elsewhere, and in one it was unclear.[31] Forty-seven were funded exclusively by pharmaceutical companies, ten by government research institutes with or without supplementary pharmaceutical support, and funding for three studies was not reported.[28, 32, 33] All studies enrolled both men and women except one VA study which enrolled only men.[30] Among the RCTs, most enrolled a broad age range of patients from age 18 to no upper age limit; only three had a lower age limit of 40.[3, 5, 30] As shown in Appendix E, Table 1 there was a wide spectrum of hypoglycemic treatment regimens and of other inclusion criteria.

Definition of Severe Hypoglycemia

All 60 studies met our pre-specified minimal definition of severe hypoglycemia: an episode with typical symptoms (e.g., sweating, dizziness, tremor, visual disturbance) that resolves after treatment (oral carbohydrate, intramuscular glucagon, or intravenous glucose) administered by another person. Adopting the language used in ACCORD,[3] we refer to this type of episode as **HA—Hypoglycemia needing any Assistance.** Thirty-seven studies used this definition exclusively. Six studies required that the episode be treated by medical personnel to qualify as "severe"—referred to as **HMA (Hypoglycemia requiring Medical Assistance);** ten studies used other definitions (see Appendix E, Table 1); and seven studies categorized events by more than one definition.

Study Quality

As shown in Appendix D, Table 1, only 26% (n=12) of the 46 unique randomized studies were rated as a good quality study or having a low risk of bias based on adequate allocation concealment, blinding, analysis by intent-to-treat, and adequate study withdrawal reporting. The remaining studies were assessed as fair quality with an unclear risk of bias. Adequate methods used to conceal allocation was reported in 41% (n=19) of the studies, and any blinding (participants, personnel, and/or outcome assessors) was reported in 63% (n=29) of studies. Most studies analyzed data based on randomized subjects who had taken at least one dose of study medication (modified intent-to-treat). Reasons for dropouts/attrition were generally reported. Nearly all studies reported funding from pharmaceutical industries.

Among the 14 unique non-randomized studies for Key Question #1, eight were prospective cohort studies, five were retrospective cohort studies and one was a case series (Appendix D, Table 2). Although our intent was to exclude case series, this study was originally misclassified and was retained in our analysis. Most studies used a study sample that pertained to the population of interest, included inclusion/ exclusion criteria, and used appropriate sampling methods. Outcomes reporting and measurement assessment were considered appropriate in nearly all studies. Methods for minimizing confounding were reported in seven of the studies.

Results

We tabulated frequency of severe hypoglycemia by treatment regimen (Appendix E, Table 3). Overall incidence of severe hypoglycemia was low in most studies, particularly studies of metformin monotherapy(<1%), GLP-1 analogs (< 1%), DPP-4 inhibitors (<1%), glinides (0%), detemir (<1%) and TZDs (<1%). In the single study evaluating pramlintide, the incidence of severe hypoglycemia was less than 2%, the same as the placebo incidence.[34] We pooled incidence data for specific treatment regimens as detailed below.

Long-acting Insulins

There were eight studies of <u>insulin glargine</u>,[35-42] three long term (pooled incidence 4.1%, 95% CI 1.9 to 8.4%, N=1223) and five short-term (pooled incidence 1.6%, 95% CI 0.8 to 3.2%, N=13,088) (Appendix F, Figure 1). There were three <u>insulin detemir</u> studies[18, 40, 43] (Appendix F, Figure 2), two long-term (incidence 1.4%, 95% CI 0.7 to 2.9%, N=525) and one moderate term (incidence 0.4%, 95% CI 0.1 to 0.9%, N=1129). <u>NPH insulin monotherapy</u> was studied in two trials[35, 39] (Appendix F, Figure 3), with a pooled incidence of 9.3% (95% CI 7.3 to 11.8%, N=763) over a weighted average follow-up time of 3.5 years. Six studies with eight treatment arms evaluated <u>NPH insulin in combination with other glucose lowering medications</u>[35, 39, 41, 44-46] (Appendix F, Figure 4). Five of the six studies were short-term and one was long-term. Pooled incidence was 5.0% (95% CI 4.1 to 6.1%, N=3150) over a weighted average follow-up time of 1.2 years. We also pooled relative risks for <u>NPH versus glargine</u> (Appendix F, Figure 5). For this comparison there were three trials,[35, 39, 41] one long term and two short-term. There was no difference in risk over a weighted average follow-up time of 2.5 years, (RR 1.37, 95% CI 0.66 to 2.81, N=2291)

Fast-acting Insulin Analogues

In the two <u>lispro</u> studies,[36, 47] the pooled incidence of severe hypoglycemia was 3.6% (95% CI 2.3 to 5.4%, N=1198, Appendix F, Figure 6) over a weighted average follow-up time of 1.3 years. In the four studies of <u>aspart</u>,[15, 22, 43, 48] the pooled incidence of severe hypoglycemia was 0.2% (95% CI 0.2% to 0.2%, N=54,225, Appendix F, Figure 7) over a weighted average follow-up time of 0.5 years. In the 2 studies of <u>glulisine</u> (combined with NPH insulin),[45, 46] the incidence of severe hypoglycemia was 1.0% (95% CI 0.5 % to 2.1%, N=883, Appendix F, Figure 8) over a weighted average follow-up time of 0.5 years.

In the 13 <u>sulfonylurea studies</u> (Appendix F, Figure 9), the pooled incidence of severe hypoglycemia was 1.2% (95% CI 0.9 to 1.5%, N=9081) over a weighted average follow-up time of 2.3 years.[17, 18, 21, 32, 49-57]

Insulin Provision versus Insulin Sensitization

One multinational factorial trial enrolled 2307 patients with type 2 diabetes and coronary heart disease and randomized them to either a percutaneous or surgical revascularization procedure and to either an insulin sensitization (metformin and TZDs most commonly used) or an insulin provision strategy (insulin and sulfonylureas most commonly used). The target HbA1c in both groups was less than 7%. The average length of follow-up was 5.3 years. The incidence of severe hypoglycemia was 5.9% in the insulin sensitization group and 9.2% in the insulin provision group[58] (Appendix F, Figure 10).

Placebo

Two short-term (24 weeks) studies had a placebo only arm[59, 60] and one long-term (10 years) study had a diet-only arm[21, 29] with a total of 1312 subjects followed for a weighted average time of 7 years. The incidence of severe hypoglycemia was 0.6% (95% CI 0.3 to 1.2%). The two studies with placebo arms had rates of 0%.

Trials of Intensive versus Conventional Glycemic Control

Five trials randomized participants to intensive glycemic control versus conventional control[3-5, 21, 29, 30] (Table 1, below). Length of follow-up ranged from 2.3 to 10 years, with a weighted average follow-up time of 5.2 years. The pooled incidence of severe hypoglycemia in these 5 trials was 7.6% in the intensive group and 3.1% in the conventional group (RR 2.4, 95% CI 1.8 to 3.1, N= 27,644, Appendix F, Figure 11).

The largest of these trials was ACCORD[3] which enrolled over 10,000 patients in the US and Canada and randomized them to receive intensive (target HbA1c <6%) or conventional (target HbA1c 7-7.9%) treatment. This trial was stopped early due to an increase in all-cause mortality in the intensively treated group. Although this group had a higher incidence of serious hypoglycemia requiring medical assistance (which might have explained the increased mortality), subsequent analyses did not confirm an association between hypoglycemia and increased mortality.[61] The other four trials did not find increased all-cause mortality in the intensively treated arms. This discrepancy may be explained by the fact that ACCORD[3] was the largest of these trials and enrolled a higher risk population. For example, in ADVANCE,[4] the next largest trial, fewer than 2% of subjects were on insulin at baseline compared to 35% of subjects in ACCORD. Similarly, average duration of diabetes and baseline level of HbA1c were higher in ACCORD than ADVANCE.

Table 1. Incidence of Severe Hypoglycemia – Trials of Intensive vs. Conventional Glycemic Control

Study	Standard	Intensive	Average Follow-up (Years)	Definition	Glycemic Targets (conventional /intense)
ACCORD[3]	261/5123 (5.1%)	830/5128 (16.2%)	3.5	HA	HbA1c 7.0 – 7.9/ HbA1c < 6.0
ADVANCE[4]	81/5569 (1.5%)	150/5571 (2.7%)	5.0	HA	Local standards/HbA1c ≤ 6.5
VA-DT[5]	28/899 (3.1%)	76/892 (8.5%)	5.6	**	HbA1c < 9/HbA1c < 6
VA-CSDM[30]	2/78 (2.6%)	5/75 (6.6%)	2.3	HA	HbA1c < 13/HbA1c 4.0 – 6.1
UKPDS[#21, 29]	8/1138 (0.7%)	33/3071 (1.1%)	10.0	HA	FPG 6.1 – 15.0 mmol/l/ FPG < 6.0 mmol/l

** life threatening or resulted in death, hospitalization, disability or incapacity
 # data for the 2 UKPDS studies are combined as per Hemmingsen 2011[9]
HA—episode of hypoglycemia requiring assistance of another person

Other Meta-Analyses

We identified four high quality meta-analyses comparing intensive versus conventional control strategies.[8-11] These reviews reported a 2- to 2.5- fold increased risk of severe hypoglycemia in intensively treated patients, with 5 year incidence rates of 2-3% with conventional control and 5-7% with intensive control. In addition, several high quality reviews have pooled data on specific diabetes treatments including exenatide,[62, 63] sitagliptin,[64] long-acting insulin analogs,[65, 66] fast acting insulin analogs,[67, 68] liragultide,[63] insulin with or without oral hypoglycemic agents (OHAs),[69] insulin with pioglitzone[70] and glinides.[71] As shown in Table 2, the frequency of severe hypoglycemia was less than1% in all these reviews.

Table 2. Frequency of Severe Hypoglycemia in Prior Reviews

Treatment	Reference	# of Studies*	Frequency of Severe Hypoglycemia
Exenatide	Waugh[62]	7	Rare episodes, mostly when combined with sulfonylureas
	Shyangdan[63]	3	1 episode
Sitagliptin	Richter[64]	11	0 episodes
Glargine, Detemir (long acting insulin analogs)	Swinnen[65]	4	No difference between determir and glargine
	Horvath[66]	4	No difference between analogs and NPH
Lispro, Glulisine, Aspart (fast acting insulin analogs)	Siebenhofer[67]	14	Incidence ranged from 0 to 30.3 (median 0.3) episodes per 100 pt-yrs compared to 0-50.4 (median 1.4) per 100 pt-yrs for people on regular insulin
	Tran[68]	2	No difference between Lispro 2/811 (0.1%) and Human Insulin 5/811 (0.6%)
Liragultide	Shyangdan[63]	3 (1.2 mg) 4 (1.8 mg)	1.2 mg dose: 0 episodes; 1.8 mg dose: 6 episodes
Insulin with or without OHA	Goudsward[69]	14	1 episode
Insulin with Pioglitazone	Clar[70]	6	"severe hypoglycemia rarely seen"
Glinides	Black[71]	5	4 studies had 0 episodes; 1 study (repaglinide) had 3 episodes (1%)

reporting severe hypoglycemia

Extension of Key Question #1

In order to gain a more population-based perspective on hypoglycemia incidence, we re-reviewed all the abstracts identified through the initial search strategy (through November 2011) to find articles that might contain data from more representative groups that had not met the initial inclusion criteria (see Methods). From this search we identified 16 additional studies.

Overview of Included Studies

The 16 studies included 13 cross-sectional patient surveys, retrospective analyses of administrative data, and 1 prospective cohort study.[72] Six of the studies were from the US, nine from Europe, and one from Asia.[73] Ten were funded in whole or in part by industry, two by the VA,[74, 75] three by foundations or other government agencies,[76-78] and funding was not reported for one study.[79] For more details on these studies see Appendix E, Table 2.

Patient Surveys (n=13)

Six reported events from the previous 6 months,[73, 74, 78, 80-83] five from the previous year,[76-79, 84] one from the previous 5 years[85] and one from the previous 2 weeks.[86] Seven studies included patients on any OHA, three on insulin only, two on a SU with or without metformin, and one on any combination of medications.[79] Eleven studies categorized hypoglycemic events as requiring assistance from another person (six further categorized events as requiring medical (HMA) or non-medical assistance (HA)) and two had other definitions.[80, 86] Sample sizes ranged from 215 to 5965.

All the survey studies which had 6 months of follow-up and reported severe hypoglycemia included patients on OHA only.[73, 74, 82, 83, 87] In these five studies rates of HA were 1%, 2%, 4%, 9%, and 13% and of HMA were 2%,[83] 1%,[82] 4%,[87] and 3%.[73] In the three of the four studies with 1 year of follow-up,[76, 77, 84] all of which included patients on insulin only, rates of HA were 12, 15 and 17 % and of HMA 2% (Honkasalo et al.[77] only study to report). The four remaining survey studies included one in which 14% of 2074 patients on OHA only reported one or more symptomatic episodes (not necessarily severe) in past 2 weeks;[86] one in which 27% of 1709 patients on OHA reported HA and 5% reported HMA over past 5 years;[85] one in which symptomatic hypoglycemia (not necessarily severe) occurred in the previous 6 months in 20% of 203 patients;[80] and one in which 27% of 635 people on insulin and 6% of 2689 people on OHA only reported HA in one year.[79]

Results from Other Studies (n=3)

- In a community based study in Scotland, a random sample of 173 adults with type 2 diabetes prospectively recorded hypoglycemic episodes over 1 month. Five (3%) experienced one or more severe episodes (required the assistance of another person).[72]

- In a US study using claims data from a privately insured population of adults age less than 65 with type 2 diabetes on either glargine (N=400) or NPH (N=400), 0.75% in each group had one or more hypoglycemia related outpatient claims during 1 year.[88]

- In a retrospective cohort analysis of 243,222 VA patients, diabetic patients with chronic kidney disease (CKD) had an average of 2.99 hypoglycemic events (glucose < 50) per 100 patient-months compared to 1.45 events in those without chronic kidney disease.[75]

Summary of Key Question #1

Overall incidence of severe hypoglycemia was less than 1% in the majority of the 60 reviewed studies, particularly those of metformin monotherapy (<1%), GLP-1 analogs (<1%), DPP-4 inhibitors (<1%), insulin detemir (<1%), insulin aspart (<1%), glinides (0%) and TZDs (<1%). The data suggest annual rates of severe hypoglycemia greater than 1% for NPH, glargine, lispro, glulisine and sulfonylureas. Some of the highest rates of severe hypoglycemia were observed in the intensive control arms of large trials comparing this treatment to conventional control (e.g., ACCORD).

Of the additional 16 studies reviewed to gain a broader population-based perspective on incidence of symptomatic hypoglycemia, 13 were survey studies reporting patient-recalled rates. Eleven of these 13 asked patients to report on events in the past 6 months (N=6) to one year (N=5). In these 11 studies patient reported incidences of hypoglycemia varied widely from 1% to 17%.

KEY QUESTION #2. What are the risk factors for severe hypoglycemia in adults with type 2 diabetes on one or more hypoglycemic agents (e.g., demographics, co-morbidities, diabetes treatment regimen, other medication use, goal and achieved HbA1c)?

We identified 31 articles on 28 studies that provided information about risk factors for severe hypoglycemia.

Overview of Included Studies (Appendix E, Table 1)

An overview of the 31 included articles is shown in Appendix E, Table 1. These 31 articles represent 28 unique studies, including four randomized controlled trials,[43, 89-91] three prospective cohort studies (in five articles),[16, 17, 92-94] five retrospective cohort studies, [25, 95-98] seven cross sectional studies,[76, 78, 84, 85, 99-101] seven case control studies,[24, 27, 102-106] and three case series,[107, 108] one of which was related to a prospective cohort study.[17] Although we excluded case series, two studies were originally misclassified and retained in our analyses. Four studies were multinational,[3, 4, 85, 107] seven were performed in the United States, three in Germany, three in Scotland, three in the UK, and eight in other countries (Australia, Denmark, Mexico, Sweden, Italy, Japan, Greece, Poland). All of the studies enrolled both men and women. Average age ranged from the mid 50s to the low 80s, with 14 of the studies having an average age in the 60s. Six studies[17, 24, 25, 27, 43, 85, 109] were entirely funded by a pharmaceutical company. Funding for nine studies was supplied by government agencies with or without supplementary pharmaceutical company support. Funding for 13 studies was not reported.

Although all 28 studies are included in Appendix E, Tables 4 and 5, in the text below we summarize 14 articles on 12 unique study populations. Sixteen articles were not included in this summary because they did not report multivariate analyses of risk factors. One additional article was excluded since the multivariate analysis evaluated any (not severe) hypoglycemia.[24] The 12 studies included two RCTs, one prospective and one retrospective cohort, four cross sectional, and four case control studies.

Definition of Severe Hypoglycemia

All 28 studies met our pre-specified minimal definition of severe hypoglycemia as defined in Key Question #1. Of the 12 multivariate adjusted studies, four used HA (**H**ypoglycemia needing any **A**ssistance), three used HMA (**H**ypoglycemia requiring **M**edical **A**ssistance), three used administration of IV glucose, and two studies categorized events by more than one definition.[3, 92]

Quality

The quality of both RCTs was good. Of the non-randomized studies, 9 of 12 met criteria for three or more of the quality metrics (Appendix D, Table 3).

Results (See Table 3 and Appendix E, Table 6)

Since the studies varied considerably with respect to risk factors evaluated (and their definitions), populations studied, and lengths of follow-up, the data were considered unsuitable for pooling. We present, instead, a narrative summary. Although *impaired hypoglycemia awareness* was evaluated in only one study, it is frequently listed as a well-established risk factor so we include it here as well. The single study that met our criteria was a cross sectional survey of 401 subjects, in which impaired awareness was associated with an increased risk of hypoglycemia (OR 2.66, 95% CI 1.55 to 4.56).[84] The risk factor *intensive glycemic control* is discussed above under Key Question #1.

Gender was evaluated as a risk factor in seven studies,[16, 27, 89, 90, 97, 100, 102] with mixed findings. Most studies, including the large ADVANCE trial, showed no association between gender and risk for severe hypoglycemia.[16, 90, 102] One large retrospective cohort study showed that men were at higher risk than women, but the 95% confidence interval extended to 1.0.[97] In ACCORD, women were more likely than men to experience a hypoglycemic event requiring medical assistance (HR 1.21, 95% CI 1.02 to 1.43). Similarly, in a nested case-control study using a claims database, men on at least one OHA had a 16% lower risk of hypoglycemia-associated hospitalization than women (OR 0.84, 95% CI 0.73 to 0.96).[27]

Table 3. Significant Risk Factors for Severe Hypoglycemia

Study, year	Older Age	Male Gender	Nonwhite Race	Married	Advanced Education	Impaired Awareness	Alcohol	Smoking	Lower BMI	Longer Diabetes Duration	Higher HbA1c	Previous Hypoglycemia	Polypharmacy	Renal Disease	Microvascular Complications	Macrovascular complications	Dementia or cognitive impairment	Intense control	Insulin or insulin dose	Time on insulin	Metformin	Sulfonylurea or dose	Other
Akram 2006[84]****	X			↑		↑		X		↑					↑	X			X		X		↓
Bruce 2009[92]**	X	X		X					↑	X	↑	↑		↑	X	X	↑		↑	↑			↑
Davis 2010[16]**,***	X	X			↑		X		X	X	↑	↑		↑	↑				↑	↑		X	↑
Davis 2011[93]**	X	X			↑		X		X	X	X	↑	X	↑	↑				X	↑		X	↑
Duran-Nah 2008[104]	↓				↓					↑		↑		↑									↑
Holstein 2009[102]	↓	X							X	X	X		X	X		↑	X		X		X	↑	
Holstein 2011[103]											↓		X										↑
Miller 2001[100]******	X	X	X						X	X	X	X		X					X			X	X
Miller 2010[89]	↑	↓	↓↑*****		↓		X		↑	↑*	↑			↑	↑	X		↑	↑		↓	X	↓
Quilliam 2011[27]	X	↓										↑		↑	↑	↑			↑			↑	↑
Sarkar 2010[78]*******	X	X	X		↓		X		X	X	X			X	X	X	X		X		X	X	
Shen 2008[101]********	X	X	↑														X						
Shorr 1997[97]	↑	↑	↑				↑			↑			↑						↑			↑	
Zoungas 2010[90]	↑	X			↓			↑	↑	↑	X			↑	↑	X	↑	↑			X		↑

↑ = significantly increase the risk of hypoglycemia in multivariate analysis
↓ = significantly decrease the risk of hypoglycemia in multivariate analysis
X = risk factors included in the multivariate model AND non significant risk factors
Microvascular Disease: microalbuminuria, diabetic eye disease, peripheral neuropathy
Macrovascular Disease: stroke, transient ischemic attack, myocardial infarction, angina, coronary or peripheral revascularization, leg amputation
* Total time since diagnosis of diabetes not significant, but 16+ years ↑
**Data from Fremantle Diabetes Study
*** compiled data from all multivariate models
**** includes both any event and repeated events
***** ↑ for African American, ↓ for "Other"
****** Includes intensive, standard, and combined
******* Only evaluated one risk factor as independent variable

Race was evaluated in four studies, three of which found that blacks are at higher risk for severe hypoglycemia than whites. These studies included one large RCT,[89] two retrospective cohort studies,[97, 100] and one cross-sectional study.[101] ACCORD reported that, compared to non-Hispanic whites, blacks had a 43% increased risk of HMA (HR 1.43, 95% CI 1.2 to 1.7) and that people in racial groups other than Hispanic or black had a lower risk of HMA than whites (HR 0.64, 95% CI 0.47 to 0.88).[89] An increased risk for African Americans was also seen in a large population-based retrospective cohort study of 20,000 Medicaid enrollees over age 65 in Tennessee. Specifically, blacks on OHAs had a two-fold increased risk of hypoglycemia-related hospitalization, ED visit or death compared to whites (RR 2.0, 95% CI 1.7 to 2.4).[97] A cross-sectional analysis of hospitalizations among people with type 2 diabetes in US community hospitals indicated that blacks were more likely than whites to have a diagnosis of acute hypoglycemic condition (OR 1.62, 95% CI 1.55 to 1.69).[101]

Body mass index was evaluated in five studies, including two large RCTS,[89, 90] both of which found that a higher BMI was associated with a lower risk of severe hypoglycemia. In ACCORD,[89] a BMI of 30 or higher was associated with a 35% lower incidence of HMA than a BMI of less than 25 (HR 0.65, 95% CI 0.5 to 0.85). Similarly, in ADVANCE[90] for each unit (kg/m^2) increase in BMI there was a 5% decrease in risk of HA (HR 0.95, 95% CI 0.93 to 0.98). BMI was not found to be associated with risk in three smaller studies.[16, 100, 102]

Age was evaluated as a risk factor for severe hypoglycemia in nine studies (two RCTs, one prospective and one retrospective cohort, one cross sectional, and four case control). The two largest trials (ACCORD[89] and ADVANCE[90]) both reported significant associations between older age and risk of severe hypoglycemia. In ACCORD,[89] the risk of HMA increased by 3% for each additional year of age (HR 1.03, 95% CI 1.02 to 1.05). ADVANCE[90] reported almost identical results (HR 1.05, 95% CI 1.03 to 1.07). Confirming these findings, a population-based retrospective cohort study of 20,000 Medicaid enrollees over age 65 in Tennessee, found that compared to enrollees age 65-69, older age groups had significantly increased risk (age 70-74: RR 1.1, 95% CI 0.9 to 1.4; age 75-79: RR 1.5, 95% CI 1.2 to 1.9; age ≥ 80: RR 1.8, 95% CI 1.4 to 2.3).[97] Six smaller studies showed either no significant association between age and risk of severe hypoglycemia[16, 27, 84, 100] or a significant <u>inverse</u> association.[102, 104]

Diabetes duration was evaluated as a risk factor in seven studies (two RCTs, one prospective and one retrospective cohort, two case control, one cross sectional). In ACCORD, compared to people with diabetes duration of 5 years or less, the risk for those with diabetes duration of 11-15 years increased by a non-significant 6% (HR 1.06, 95% CI 0.83 to 1.37) and by 37% for those with diabetes of 16 or more years (HR 1.37, 95% CI 1.09 to 1.73).[89] In ADVANCE each year of diabetes was associated with a 2% increase in risk of severe hypoglycemia (HR 1.02, 95% CI 1.00 to 1.04).[90] Similar results were reported by the cross sectional[84] and one of the case control studies.[104] The other three studies did not find statistically significant associations between duration of diabetes and incidence of severe hypoglycemia.[16, 100, 102]

Previous hypoglycemia was evaluated as a risk factor in four studies, two case control,[27, 104] one prospective,[16] and one retrospective cohort.[100] Three studies found that a history of past hypoglycemia was a strong predictor of future episodes, and one did not.[100] In a large case control study based on administrative data, a prior emergency room (ER) visit for hypoglycemia increased the odds of a subsequent inpatient admission for hypoglycemia by more than nine-fold (OR 9.5, 95% CI 5 to 18).[27] In the other case control study a reported history of hypoglycemia, not further defined, in the previous year was associated with a three-fold increase risk of hypoglycemia associated hospitalization or ER visit (OR 2.9, 95% CI 1.3 to 6.5).[104] History of previous episode requiring health services use was associated with a six-fold increase for another episode over the next 8 years (HR 5.7, 95% CI 2.2 to 15) in the prospective cohort study.[16]

Education was evaluated as a risk factor in five studies, two RCTS,[89, 90] one cross sectional,[78] one case control[104] and one prospective cohort study.[16] Four of the five studies found significant but modest associations between level of education and risk for severe hypoglycemia. ADVANCE found a marginally significant inverse association between the age at completion of formal education and risk of severe hypoglycemia (HR 0.98 95% CI 0.96 to 1.0).[90] Similarly, in ACCORD, subjects with less than a high school education were at an increased risk for severe hypoglycemia (conventional control: HR 1.74, 95% CI 1.02 to 2.95; intensive control: HR 1.38, 95% CI 1.06 to 1.81) compared to those with more education.[89] In the case control study, illiteracy was associated with an increased risk (OR 3.7, 95% CI 1.4 to 10).[104] In a cross sectional study in a community population, Sarkar et al. found that subjects who indicated that they had "problems learning," "needed help reading," or "lacked confidence with forms" were about 30-40% more likely to have reported an HA in the previous year.[78] Finally, in the prospective cohort study, "education level higher than primary level" was associated with an increased risk of severe hypoglycemia (HR 2.3, 95% CI 1.09 to 5.04, N=616).[16]

Renal disease was evaluated as a risk factor in seven studies, two RCTs,[89, 90] one prospective,[16] one retrospective cohort[100] study, and three case control studies.[27, 102, 104] Five of these studies found that renal insufficiency (defined as elevated serum creatinine level or elevated estimated glomerular filtration rate) was significantly associated with increased risk of severe hypoglycemia. The only studies that did not find a significant association were a very small study,[102] and the retrospective cohort study that was conducted in a single institution with a predominantly African American population.[100] In ACCORD, a urine albumin:creatinine ratio greater than 300 or a serum creatinine greater than 115 umol/L were each associated with a significantly increased risk of about 70%. In ADVANCE, for each umol/L increase in serum creatinine, the risk of a severe hypoglycemic event increased by 1%.[90]

Other (non-renal) microvascular disease was assessed in five studies.[16, 27, 84, 89, 90] In four of the five there were significant positive associations; in one relatively small study (N=415), which evaluated untreated retinopathy and symptomatic or asymptomatic peripheral neuropathy, there were no statistically significant associations for any event, but peripheral neuropathy was found in increase the risk of repeated events of severe hypoglycemia.[84] In ACCORD a history of peripheral neuropathy conferred a modest but significant increased risk (HR 1.2, 95% CI 1.1 to 1.4).[89] In ADVANCE a "history of microvascular disease" conferred a twofold increased risk of severe hypoglycemia (HR 2.1, 95% CI 1.5 to 3.).[90] In a nested case-control database study, peripheral ulceration was found to be positively associated with risk of inpatient hospital admission for hypoglycemia (OR 1.71, 95% CI 1.2 to 2.44).[27] Finally a population based but relatively small study (N=616) found that a history of peripheral neuropathy was significantly associated with severe hypoglycemia (HR 2.4, 95% CI 1.3 to 4.5).[16]

Dementia was evaluated as a risk factor for severe hypoglycemia in three studies.[90, 92, 103] In ADVANCE, higher cognitive function as measured by the Mini Mental Status Examination was significantly associated with a modest decreased risk of severe hypoglycemia (HR 0.93, 95% CI 0.87 to 0.99).[90] In the second study, which was population based and prospectively followed 302 patients age 70 years and older, patients with dementia at baseline had a significantly higher risk for hypoglycemia requiring medical attention than those who did not have dementia (HR 3.0, 95% CI 1.1 to 8.5).[92] In a small case control study, dementia was not found to be a significant risk factor.[103]

Other risk factors evaluated in the 12 studies included genetic markers, marital status, smoking, alcohol consumption, polypharmacy, recent discharge from the hospital, and use of ACE inhibitors. All were found, in one or more studies, to be associated with increased risk of hypoglycemia (See Appendix D, Table 6). However, these findings were generally sparse, often conflicting, and ultimately inconclusive.

Summary of Key Question #2

Factors most consistently and independently associated with risk for severe hypoglycemia in adult patients with type 2 diabetes on hypoglycemic medication include: intensive glycemic control (discussed above under Key Question #1), history of hypoglycemia, renal insufficiency, history of microvascular complications, longer diabetes duration, lower education level, African American race and history of dementia. History of hypoglycemia unawareness was evaluated in only one study. Gender, age and lower BMI were not consistently associated with risk, although higher age and lower BMI were associated with higher risk in the two largest studies.

KEY QUESTION #3. What is the effect of severe hypoglycemia on other outcomes in adults with type 2 diabetes on one or more hypoglycemic agents (e.g., quality of life, mortality, morbidity, utilization)?

We identified 59 articles on 53 studies that provided information about outcomes in patients who experienced severe hypoglycemia.

Overview of Included Studies (Appendix E, Table 1)

An overview of the 59 included articles is provided in Appendix E, Table 1. Among the 53 studies were 14 randomized controlled trials,[3-5, 21, 30, 41, 42, 46, 52, 54, 110-113] 16 cohort studies,[17, 19, 25, 26, 75, 92, 94-97, 114-118] 12 cross sectional studies,[78, 81, 82, 99, 119-126] and 11 case control or case series studies.[9, 28, 105, 107-109, 127-131] Twelve studies were multinational; additionally, twelve were performed in the United States, four in Germany, three in the UK, three in Scotland, three in Sweden, and the remainder in other countries (Canada, Australia, Singapore, India, Israel, Netherlands, Turkey, Switzerland, France, Italy, Greece, and Poland). All but one of the studies[30] enrolled both men and women. Average age ranged from 30 to 85 years with most studies reporting a mean age in the 50 or 60 year range. Twenty one studies were entirely funded by a pharmaceutical company while eight studies were funded by government agencies, three by private foundations, and five by multiple funding sources. No source of funding was listed for 16 studies.

All-Cause Mortality

All-cause mortality associated with severe hypoglycemia was reported in three large randomized trials that compared intensive control to conventional control.[3, 4, 21, 61, 90] Mortality ranged from zero to 12.5 percent in intensively treated people who became hypoglycemic; in two of these three studies mortality in this group was 0.1% or less and in the third there was one death in eight study subjects (12.5%). In all three randomized trials, mortality in the conventional control groups ranged from 0% to 1.2%.

Six additional randomized trials (typically fewer than 1,000 patients enrolled with follow-up less than 30 weeks) compared different treatment regimens, including oral medications and different forms of insulin.[42, 43, 46, 52, 111-113] No deaths related to severe hypoglycemia were reported in these studies.

Eight cohort studies reported mortality outcomes, typically in patients seen in an ER or hospitalized for severe hypoglycemia. There were no deaths in three studies.[16, 17, 116] In four other studies, between 0.3% and 8.3% of the patients died following severe hypoglycemic events.[95-97,98] One study of veterans with and without CKD did not report number of deaths but reported odds ratios for outpatient risk of death within one day of a hypoglycemic event (defined as glucose <50 mg/dl) compared to individuals with glucose of ≥70 mg/dl.[75] For patients without CKD, the odds ratio was 13.28 (95% CI 9.30 to 19.18). For patients with CKD, the odds ratio was 6.84 (95% CI 4.41 to 10.62).

Mortality was also assessed in six case series. As with the cohort studies, these studies also enrolled patients seen in an emergency room or admitted to a hospital as a result of severe hypoglycemia. Four studies reported no deaths.[28, 108, 109, 128] Three other studies reported that between 3.2% and 11% of the enrolled patients died after severe hypoglycemia.[105, 127, 131]

Three studies reported long-term follow-up mortality data. Participants in the ADVANCE trial were followed for a median of 5 years.[90] The mortality rate was 19.5% in those who had experienced at least one episode of severe hypoglycemia and 9.0% in those who had not (adjusted HR 3.27, 95% CI 2.29 to 4.65). The median time to death was 1.05 years. In a prospective cohort study, there were no deaths at the time of the event but 16 of the 45 patients (35.6%) died during the mean follow-up period of 22.8 months.[17] The third study, a retrospective cohort study that observed in-hospital mortality of 1.6% (2 of 126 patients), reported long-term mortality of 42.1% (53 of 126 patients) during a median follow-up of 23.2 months. Of the 53 total deaths, 20 were in the group of patients treated with oral medications and 33 were in the group treated with insulin (univariate analysis, p=0.02).[95] The authors reported that median annual mortality in the study population was 22% and compared that to 5.2% in the general population (patients with and without diabetes, age 80 years).

Non-fatal Myocardial Infarction

Three randomized trials, one cohort study, and one case series provided information about non-fatal myocardial infarctions among patients with severe hypoglycemia. Two randomized trials reported no events.[30, 113] The third reported that one patient (4.5%) experienced severe hypoglycemia with cardiac arrest.[110] The authors did not say how much time elapsed between the hypoglycemic episodes and the cardiac arrests. A cohort study that enrolled individuals who experienced severe hypoglycemia reported three cases (0.5%) with myocardial infarction as a complication of the hypoglycemia.[97] A case series reported two cases (2%) of transient asymptomatic myocardial ischemia associated with severe hypoglycemia.[127]

Non-fatal Stroke

Non-fatal stroke outcomes were reported in four studies. A randomized trial of several hypoglycemic therapies reported no stroke events.[113] A cohort study with 586 patients reported seven patients (1.2%) experiencing stroke as a complication of severe hypoglycemia.[97] A case series of 207 patients admitted to a hospital with severe hypoglycemia during a three year period, included two patients (0.97%) who experienced cerebrovascular ischemic stroke.[108] In a case series of 19 patients with severe hypoglycemia associated with glipizide use (over a 7 year period), one patient (5.3%) who had a stroke prior to the hypoglycemic event experienced further functional impairment. The patient died 23 days after the event.[105]

Other Neurologic Events

Two randomized trials with veterans assigned to either intensive or conventional control reported data on other neurologic events associated with severe hypoglycemia. In one trial, loss of consciousness was reported for both of the conventional control group patients who experienced severe hypoglycemia (2.6% of the conventional control group) and none of the five intensive control patients who experienced severe hypoglycemia (0% of the intensive control group).[30] In the second trial, severe hypoglycemia with impaired consciousness was reported in three episodes/100 patient-years in the conventional control group compared to nine episodes/100 patient-years in the intensive control group. In addition, complete loss of consciousness was reported in one episode/100 patient-years and three episodes/100 patient-years, respectively. Both differences were significant (p<0.001). The median follow-up in the trial was 5.6 years.[5]

Five randomized trials of different treatment regimens also reported neurologic outcomes. Two trials reported zero events.[41, 54] In another trial, at the three year follow-up, loss of consciousness associated with severe hypoglycemia was reported by four patients – one in the biphasic aspart group (0.4%) and three in the basal detemir group (1.3%).[43] One trial reported one patient with a coma (0.5%) among 199 treated with NPH plus regular human insulin.[112] In the last trial, seven episodes in four patients either required medical assistance or were accompanied by neurological symptoms.[52]

Three cohort studies provided data on neurologic outcomes. One study reported that, at presentation to a hospital, 51% were in a coma, 18% were disoriented, 11% experienced somnolence, 9% experienced paralysis, 7% had cerebral seizures and 5% had psychological disturbances.[17] In another study, among 126 patients admitted for severe hypoglycemia, 54% of oral hypoglycemic agent users experienced coma compared to 30.2% of insulin users.[95] A third study reported transient ischemic attack as a complication of severe hypoglycemia in four patients (0.7%).[97] At presentation, a loss of consciousness was observed in 49% of episodes, seizures in 5% of episodes and irrational behavior in 6% of episodes.[97]

Seven other studies reported on this outcome. A cross-sectional study reported that 4% of patients experienced convulsions associated with episodes of severe hypoglycemia in the past year.[99] In five case series, coma was reported in 19% to 71% of individuals with severe hypoglycemia.[105, 107, 108, 128] "Semi-coma" (30%),[108] coma or stupor (21%),[28] somnolence (51%),[128] decreased consciousness (16%),[105] seizures (8-10%),[107, 127] disorientation (81%),[107] and transient right hemiplegia (1%)[127] were also reported. One study documented seizures and/or psychological disturbances in 30% of patients with severe hypoglycemia.[128]

Hospitalization

Five randomized trials reported hospitalization data. One trial of intensive versus conventional control among veterans reported no hypoglycemia-associated hospitalizations.[30] Four trials of different treatment regimens found between 0%[41, 42, 113, 132] and 0.8%[112] were hospitalized for hypoglycemia.

Hospitalizations were also reported in nine cohort studies (10 papers). Among patients starting insulin, there were no hospitalizations in 9970 patient years of observation.[26] A study of 344 veterans followed for one year identified 55 severe hypoglycemic episodes in 19 subjects; two of these (3.6%) required hospitalization.[19] A mean hospitalization rate of 0.15 episode/patient/year was reported for type 2 patients based on data from 21 patients with 29 severe hypoglycemic episodes.[116] A hospitalization rate of 47 per 1000 person-years was reported based on data from all discharges from Navajo Area Indian Health Service hospitals during a 5 year period with an estimated 26,125 person-years of observation.[96] A study that included both type 1 and type 2 patients reported that over a mean follow-up of 2.5 years, insulin-treated individuals with diabetes who had hypoglycemic episodes had more overall hospital admissions (0.97 per year vs. 0.48 per year in insulin-treated individuals without hypoglycemic episodes, p<0.01). Forty percent of the excess hospital admissions were due to hypoglycemia.[118]

Three other cohort studies (four papers) reported hospitalization associated with 17% to 33% of hypoglycemic events[25, 114, 133] or 7.1% of patients experiencing hypoglycemia.[117] Another study reported that 16% of patients seen in the emergency department were subsequently admitted to the hospital.[115]

In a cross-sectional study of patients with type 2 diabetes from a large diabetes registry, 8% of the patients with a self-reported significant hypoglycemia episode had a documented emergency room visit or hospitalization. The odds of an emergency room visit or hospitalization were significantly higher in patients who reported having at least one significant hypoglycemia episode (OR 19.0, 95% CI 13.0 to 26.0) compared to those without a significant hypoglycemia episode.[78] One other cross-sectional study reported no hospitalizations[125] while a second reported that 5.5% of patients were treated in an emergency department or hospitalized following severe hypoglycemia.[124]

Length of hospital stay, reported in two case series, ranged from a median of 5.5 days[128] to means of 9.8 days for patients on oral medications and 8.0 days for patients taking insulin.[95]

Emergency Department Visits

Two randomized trials reported that no patients with severe hypoglycemia required an emergency department visit.[42, 113] A third randomized trial reported that either 0% (insulin glargine group) or 15.4% (NPH group) of those with severe hypoglycemia were seen in the emergency department.[41, 132]

Four cohort studies reported emergency department use. One study reported that between 14% and 23% of severe hypoglycemic episodes were treated in the emergency room.[114, 133] Another cohort study reported that 31% of the patients enrolled, all of whom were eventually hospitalized, were treated first in the emergency department[17] while a third found that 8% of patients were treated in either the emergency or primary care service, 36% were treated by an ambulance service and 55% required both ambulance and emergency or clinic service.[25] Finally, over a mean follow-up of 2.5 years, insulin-treated diabetic individuals who experienced hypoglycemic episodes had higher rates of overall emergency department use (0.85 visits per year vs. 0.40 visits per year in insulin-treated diabetic individuals who did not have a hypoglycemic episode, p<0.01) with 53% of the excess visits due to hypoglycemia.[118]

Two cross-sectional studies (noted above) reported on rates of either hospitalization or emergency department visit (5.5% to 8%).[78, 124] An additional cross-sectional study reported that six of the seven patients with severe hypoglycemia during a one month period required medical services including three emergency room visits.[125]

Accident/Trauma

An evidence report prepared for the Federal Motor Carrier Safety Administration (FMCSA)[134] focused on the risk of motor vehicle crashes in drivers with diabetes and the relationship with hypoglycemia. Based on data from 13 case-control studies of low to moderate quality, the conclusion was that the risk for crash among drivers with diabetes was higher than for those without diabetes (RR 1.19, 95% CI 1.08 to 1.31). Many of the studies enrolled only patients with type 1 diabetes and all but two were published before 2000. The strength of evidence was rated as weak. To look at the effect of hypoglycemia on driving ability, the review identified three studies of moderate quality, all with type 1 patients. All three involved induced hypoglycemia and simulated driving ability. Although driving ability was impaired, it was unclear which aspects of driving ability were most affected or at what level of hypoglycemia the impairments were evident. It is unknown whether data from driving simulators are predictive of crash risk in actual driving conditions.

We identified several other studies related to motor vehicle operation that were either not included in the FMCSA review or were published after the review was completed. A case-control study identified 795 drivers who were reported (typically because of a motor vehicle crash, mandatory annual review for commercial vehicle license, license suspension appeal, or notifiable medical condition) to the Ontario Ministry of Transportation Medical Advisory Board and who had an underlying diagnosis of diabetes mellitus. The type of diabetes was not reported. Among the cases (57 drivers who had a crash), 60% reported experiencing severe hypoglycemia in the past 2 years compared to 27% of the controls (738 drivers with no crash) (OR 4.07, 95% CI 2.35 to 7.04). A lower HbA1c was also associated with an increased risk of crash even after adjusting for severe hypoglycemia (OR 1.25, 95% CI 1.02 to 1.55).[129] A cross-sectional study of diabetic patients taking hypoglycemia-inducing medications found that among the 122 patients talking oral-antidiabetics (116 with type 2 diabetes, mean age 64.2 years), subjects reported two hypoglycemia-induced accidents per year driven. Among the 151 patients receiving conventional insulin therapy (109 with type 2 diabetes, mean age 59.0 years, treated with one or two injections of premixed insulin and may also be taking other oral antidiabetics), there were three hypoglycemia-induced accidents per year driven. When asked if they refrained from driving due to fear of hypoglycemia events during driving, 0.8% of the oral medication group and 4.0% of the conventional insulin therapy group responded "yes."[121]

Several studies reported on motor vehicle accidents but did not specifically relate the outcome to severe hypoglycemia. In the ACCORD study, there was no difference in incidence of motor vehicle accidents in which the patient was the driver (0.2% in intensive therapy, 0.3% in standard therapy, p=0.40).[3] A nested case-control study used an insurance registry of all eligible drivers ages 67 to 84 years, an accident report file, and a prescription drug database. The type of diabetes was not reported. Several medication regimens were associated with a borderline significant risk of an accident. A combination of sulfonylureas and metformin was used during the preceding month by 1.6% of those involved in a crash and 1.2% of the controls (adjusted rate ratio 1.3, 95% CI 1.0 to 1.7). The adjusted rate ratio for any insulin use was 1.3 (95% CI 1.0 to 1.8). A dose-response effect was noted for users of a combination of sulfonylureas and metformin over the year preceding the index event.[135]

Six studies reported falls and bone injury data.[17, 95, 97-99, 127] A cohort study of 45 patients with sulfonylurea-induced hypoglycemia requiring hospitalization reported that six (13%) had soft tissue injuries or fractures as a result of falls associated with hypoglycemia.[17] A second cohort study of 126 type 2 diabetic patients hospitalized for severe hypoglycemia found that the percentage of patients who had experienced a fall was 21.5% with no difference between oral medication and insulin users.[95] In a third cohort study, among patients hospitalized for severe hypoglycemia, bone injuries were reported in 7.3% of patients (9.9% of the insulin users, 0% of the oral medication users).[98] A cohort study[97] and a cross-sectional study[99] reported "injury" in 1.7% to 5% of patients who experienced severe hypoglycemia. In a case series brain trauma and skeletal injury were reported in 7% of patients.[127]

Quality of Life

Nine cross-sectional studies reported measures of quality of life. One study assessed health-related quality of life with the SF-36 and reported that scores for all domains were lowest for patients reporting severe hypoglycemia.[120]

Five studies (reported in six papers) assessed health utility/quality of life with the EuroQol-5 Dimensions (EQ-5D). EQ-5D scores were lower for patients reporting severe hypoglycemia.[81, 82, 87, 119, 120, 126] Three studies reported data from the worry subscale of the Hypoglycemia Fear Survey-II (HFS-II). In two studies worry scores were highest for patients who reported severe/very severe symptoms compared to those with lesser symptoms[81, 126] while in the third study, there were no differences in worry score as severity increased.[82] Both the quality of life and the worry scores were impacted by the frequency of severe hypoglycemia episodes.[87]

Two studies looked at anxiety and depression associated with severe hypoglycemia.[122, 123] In one study, affective disorder, but not anxiety disorder, was found to be associated with a history of severe hypoglycemia in the prior 12 months.[122] The second study found that a lifetime history of at least one episode of severe hypoglycemia was associated with symptoms of anxiety (p<0.001) but not depression.[123]

Lifestyle changes made following an episode of severe hypoglycemia were the focus of one study.[124] Patients reported more frequent testing of blood glucose, changes to insulin doses, greater fear of hypoglycemia, requests to have someone check on them, and additional concerns about driving.

Other Outcomes

Cognitive Decline

Cognitive decline was reported in two cohort studies. One of the studies followed patients to determine if the risk of dementia was increased in those with at least one episode of hypoglycemia requiring hospitalization or an emergency room visit.[94] Patients who had experienced at least one episode of hypoglycemia during a 22 year period were evaluated for an additional mean of 3.8 years to determine whether they developed dementia. No patient had a diagnosis of dementia, mild cognitive impairment or general symptom memory loss at the time of the hypoglycemic episode(s). Among 1465 patients, the incidence of dementia was higher for patients who had at least one episode of hypoglycemia than for those who had no episodes (17% vs. 10%, $p < 0.001$). The attributable risk of dementia in patients with one or more episodes of hypoglycemia was 2.4% per year (95% CI 1.7 to 3.0). In the adjusted model all patients with at least one episode of severe hypoglycemia were at increased risk for dementia (hazard ratio 1.4, 95% CI 1.3 to 1.7 for one or more episodes).

In the second prospective study, a baseline assessment (the Mini-Mental State Examination and the Informant Questionnaire for Cognitive Decline in the Elderly) was completed on 302 patients age 70 and over. At 18 months, a repeat assessment was done on 205 patients (29 had died, 27 had developed dementia and 41 declined the assessment). Thirty-three new cases of cognitive decline were identified (four cases of dementia and 29 cases of cognitive impairment without dementia). There was no significant difference in prior severe hypoglycemia (either self-reported or requiring medical assistance) between those who developed cognitive decline and those who did not.[92]

Productivity

One cohort study and two cross-sectional studies reported on productivity. In the cohort study, insulin-treated patients with a medical claim coded for hypoglycemia were more likely to use short-term disability (47% vs. 32%, $p < 0.01$) and to use more sick days (19.5 vs. 11.0, $p < 0.01$) than insulin-treated patients with no claim for hypoglycemia. The analysis included patients with either type 1 or type 2 diabetes.[118] In one cross-sectional study, a mean loss of 8.6 productive days following hypoglycemia was reported for patients who experienced severe hypoglycemia; for those with mild or moderate hypoglycemia, the mean days lost was 2.7. In multivariate modeling, severity of hypoglycemia (along with frequency) was a significant predictor of productivity.[120] A second study reported that 32% of patients who experienced severe hypoglycemia went home from school, work or other activities and 26% stayed home the next day.[124]

Medical Resource Use

Several studies reported on medical service use other than hospitalization or emergency room visits. A randomized trial reported that one of five patients on liraglutide (20%) who experienced severe hypoglycemia required medical assistance of some type.[54] One cohort study reported that 1.9% of the 2,417 patients studied required medical contact for hypoglycemia during the first year of insulin use. The number decreased to 0.4% by the fourth year of use.[26] A cross-sectional study reported mean total resource use of 13.2 contacts with a health service provider among patients who reported severe hypoglycemia. For patients with mild or moderate hypoglycemia, the mean was 11.5 contacts.[120] A second cross-sectional study reported eight nurse visits, three physician visits and one telephone contact with medical care among six patients who experienced severe hypoglycemia in a one-month period (number of events not reported).[125] Another cross-sectional study reported that 2.5% of the patients experiencing severe hypoglycemia had additional visits to their physicians while 0.4% had additional communication (non-visit).[124] Two studies[114, 133] that reported hypoglycemic events before and after conversion to a pen device reported significantly fewer physician visits (37.7% of hypoglycemic events before, 28.1% after; OR 0.39, 95% CI 0.24 to 0.64), no significant difference in outpatient visits (7.8% before, 12.2% after, OR 0.79, 95% CI 0.31 to 2.01), and significantly lower use of "other" (not emergency department, hospitalization, physician visits, or outpatient visits) health care resources (22.1% before, 16.5% after, OR 0.38, 95% CI 0.20 to 0.71) after conversion to the pen device.

Summary of Key Question #3

We found good evidence for an increased risk of the following outcomes in patients who have experienced severe hypoglycemia: all-cause mortality, neurological events (other than non-fatal stroke), hospital and emergency department utilization and decreased quality of life. Severe hypoglycemia does not appear to be associated with short-term mortality. However, a history of severe hypoglycemia may contribute to increased long-term mortality. Neurological events, including coma, impaired consciousness, seizures and paralysis, were reported in seven randomized trials, three cohort studies and seven other studies. Few patients in the randomized trials experienced coma or loss of consciousness. However, in observational studies of patients presenting to an emergency department or admitted to a hospital, between 19% and 71% were in a coma. Hospitalization and emergency department utilization was reported in five randomized trials, nine cohort studies and three other studies with wide variation across studies. Although many of these studies lacked control groups, there is some evidence of increased emergency department visits and hospital admissions among patients who experience severe hypoglycemia. Data from eight cross-sectional studies suggest that patients who experience severe hypoglycemia generally report a lower quality of life and higher worry.

We found limited data about many of our outcomes of interest including non-fatal MI, non-fatal stroke, cognitive decline, motor vehicle accidents, falls and traumatic injuries, work productivity and other medical service utilization. The available evidence suggests that non-fatal MI and stroke are unlikely consequences of severe hypoglycemia. There are mixed findings from two studies on development of cognitive decline or dementia in individuals with a history of severe hypoglycemia. Few studies have reported motor vehicle accident data specifically related to severe hypoglycemia. Falls and injuries are common consequences of severe hypoglycemia but given the absence of appropriate control groups it is unclear if these outcomes are hypoglycemia-related or simply reflect the age and co-morbidity burden of the population. The evidence suggests that individuals who experience episodes of severe hypoglycemia are more likely to miss days at work. Medical resource utilization findings are difficult to interpret without appropriate control group data.

SUMMARY AND DISCUSSION

SUMMARY OF EVIDENCE BY KEY QUESTION

Key Question #1: What is the incidence of severe hypoglycemia in adults with type 2 diabetes on one or more hypoglycemic agents?

Overall incidence of severe hypoglycemia was less than 1% in the majority of the 60 reviewed studies, particularly those of metformin (0-1.5%), GLP-1 analogs (< 1%), DPP-4 inhibitors (<1%), insulin detemir (<1%), glinides (0%) and TZDs (<1%). These rates are similar to the placebo or diet-only rates which were measured in three studies[21, 29, 59, 136] with a pooled incidence of severe hypoglycemia of 0.6% (95% CI 0.3 to 1.2%) over a weighted mean follow-up time of 7 years. These results are consistent with other high quality systematic reviews of exenatide,[62, 63] liragultide,[63] sitagliptin,[64] glinides[71] and pioglitazone.[70] These results are also consistent with a recent meta-analysis of a wide variety of OHAs that concluded that severe hypoglycemia did not "occur more often with any particular monotherapy or combination therapy" but that the sulfonylureas were the most likely to increase the risk.[137] However, Bennett did not include insulins or intensive versus conventional control trials.

The treatment regimens with the highest risk were sulfonylureas, those targeting intensive control of HbA1c levels and insulin (in particular NPH, glargine, lispro, and glulisine). For the _sulfonylureas_ the pooled incidence of severe hypoglycemia was 1.2% (95% CI 0.9 to 1.5%) over a weighted average follow-up time of 2.4 years. Due to limited data we were unable to determine incidence rates associated with individual sulfonylureas.

In the five trials that randomized participants to _intensive versus conventional glycemic control_[3-5, 21, 29, 30] the pooled incidence of severe hypoglycemia was 7.6% in the intensive group and 3.1% in the conventional group (RR 2.4, 95% CI 1.8 to 3.1, N= 27,644) over a weighted average follow up of 5.2 years. This is consistent with four other high quality meta-analyses that included these RCTs and other studies and that reported a 2- to 2.5- fold increased risk of severe hypoglycemia in intensively treated patients, with 5 year incidence rates of 2-3% with conventional control and 5-7% with intensive control.[8-11] A post-hoc analysis of the ACCORD data indicated that participants whose HbA1c did not drop to target levels promptly were at the highest risk. The authors concluded that clinicians should not continue to intensify glucose lowering regimens when initial efforts are unsuccessful.[89]

Insulin

There were only two trials of _NPH monotherapy_, one of which reported a 5 year incidence of 11.1%[35] and one a 6 month incidence of 2.3%.[39] These results are consistent with two meta-analyses, one which identified no cases of severe hypoglycemia in 14 RCTs with an average follow-up of 40 weeks.[69] The second reported an incidence of severe hypoglycemia of 2.6% in six studies with 1532 subjects followed for 6 months to 1 year.[66] Overall, it appears that the annual incidence of severe hypoglycemia in persons on NPH monotherapy is about 0-3%.

For _NPH with_ OHAs we documented a pooled incidence of severe hypoglycemia of 5% (95% CI 4.1 to 6.1%, N=3150), over a weighted average followup time of 1.2 years. This is consistent with the results of a large trial in which an insulin-based strategy to lower HbA1c to less than 7% was associated with a 9.2% 5-year incidence rate[58] and another systematic review which compared long-acting insulin analogues to NPH insulin with or without concomitant OHAs and reported a 6 month 2.7% incidence of severe hypoglycemia[66] However, a review by Goudswaard,[69] which investigated either insulin monotherapy or combinations of insulin plus OHAs, identified only one severe hypoglycemic episode in a patient on morning NPH plus a sulfonylurea. In this review, 12 unique studies reported rates of hypoglycemia, none of which were included in our review because either they enrolled fewer than 500 subjects, were not published in English or were less than 6 months in duration.

Insulin detemir, a long-acting insulin analogue, was associated with a low incidence (<1%) of severe hypoglycemia, consistent with another systematic review (also including only studies of at least 6 months duration) which reported an incidence of 1.2% (7/578) in two studies.[66] However, a third review reported an incidence of severe hypoglycemia of 3.0% in four RCTs with a total of 1247 patients.[65] Since this review included studies as short as 12 weeks in duration and hypoglycemic episodes are known to occur more frequently during initiation of therapy, this may explain the discrepancy between the reviews.

Insulin glargine was evaluated in eight studies. Results from three long term studies (pooled incidence 4.1%, 95% CI 1.9 to 8.4%, N=1223) and five short-term studies (pooled incidence 1.6%, 95% CI 0.8 to 3.2%, N=13,088) are consistent with the findings of two other recent meta-analyses in which risk of severe hypoglycemia with glargine was found to be 3.2%[65] and 1.9%.[66]

Among the s*hort (or fast) acting insulin analogues (lispro, aspart, glulisine)*, for *lispro*, the pooled incidence of severe hypoglycemia was 3.6% (95% CI 2.3 to 5.4%, N=1198) over a weighted average follow-up time of 1.3 years. For *aspart*, the pooled incidence of severe hypoglycemia was 0.2% (95% CI 0.2% to 0.2%, N=54,425) over a weighted average follow-up time of 6 months; this analysis however was dominated by a very large observational study conducted in physician offices in 11 countries and funded by a pharmaceutical company.[22] If the analysis is repeated without this study the incidence is 1.5% (95% CI 0.9 to 2.5%) over a weighted mean average follow-up of years 1.2 years. For *glulisine* (combined with NPH insulin) the incidence of severe hypoglycemia was 1.0% (95% CI 0.5 % to 2.1%, N=883) over a weighted average follow-up time of 6 months.

In a meta-analysis comparing these insulins with either non-insulin agents, premixed human insulin, or long-acting insulin analogues in adults with type 2 diabetes, Qayyum found that there was no significant difference in risk of serious hypoglycemia.[138] A Canadian health technology report came to a similar conclusion, stating that there was no significant difference in severe hypoglycemia between treatment with human insulin or the insulin analogues.[68] A Cochrane review reported a median incidence of 0.3 severe hypoglycemic episodes (range 0 to 30.3) per 100 patient-years.[67] The authors attributed the wide range to the inclusion of a single study with a very short duration of follow-up.

Key Question #1 Extension

Of the additional 16 studies reviewed to gain a broader population-based perspective on incidence of severe hypoglycemia, 13 were survey studies reporting patient-recalled rates. Eleven of these asked patients to report on events in the past 6 months (N=6) to 1 year (N=5). In these 11 studies, patient reported incidences of HA varied widely from 1% to 17%. Although hypoglycemic agents are among the most commonly implicated drugs in adverse event reports and ER visits (see Key Question #3 discussion), these data do not cast any light on incidence. In the two studies least likely to be affected by recall bias, one which recorded events within the past 2 weeks[86] and the prospective study in Scotland,[72] the incidence of symptomatic hypoglycemia was 14% over 2 weeks in the former and 3% over one month in the latter. The discrepancy is likely due to Donnelly et al.'s more restrictive definition of hypoglycemia (HA as opposed to symptomatic only).

VA Specific Data

Among the studies included herein, four reported specifically on VA patients.[5, 30, 74, 75] In addition we identified two VA publications which did not meet our inclusion criteria. One was an unpublished abstract examining VA administrative data reporting that 22% of 1.4 million veterans with diabetes had a hypoglycemic associated medical encounter over 5 years. It is unclear from the abstract how the diagnoses were confirmed and what the severity of the episodes were. The second, published after our search was concluded, evaluated the incidence of hypoglycemia as determined by administrative records in 497,900 veterans aged 65 or older.[139] That study found that 7.5% of subjects had one or more inpatient or outpatient visits in which a code for hypoglycemia was recorded over 24 months.

Although suggestive of increased rates of hypoglycemia among veterans with diabetes, it is difficult to derive definitive conclusions from these VA studies since there is substantial heterogeneity with respect to definitions of hypoglycemia, study design, subject inclusion criteria, treatment regimens and lengths of follow-up.

Limitations of Available Studies

Much of the evidence comes from reports of RCTs funded by pharmaceutical companies which enroll highly selected populations and generally do not include those at highest risk for hypoglycemia. Second, the definitions of severe hypoglycemia varied among studies and there is likely substantial ascertainment bias, especially in the RCTs designed primarily to measure the benefits of specific drug regimens. Finally, there are few studies that investigated regular insulin, generally thought to be associated with high rates of hypoglycemia.

Conclusion for Key Question #1

The incidence of severe hypoglycemia is about 0-3% per year for adults with type 2 diabetes on hypoglycemic medications. Risk is highest for insulins, sulfonylureas and regimens targeting intensive control of HbA1c levels. Risk is lowest for metformin, GLP-1 analogs, DPP-4 inhibitors, glinides and TZDs. Since most of these data are derived from pharmaceutical company funded RCTS which enrolled highly selected populations, the generalizability of the results is unclear. Indeed, one small population based prospective study suggests that the incidence may be as high as 3% per month in community based subjects treated with insulin.[72] Furthermore, several studies performed in VA suggest that incidence of hypoglycemia may be higher in this population. Larger population-based prospective studies of people on a variety of hypoglycemic agents that employ accurate methods for ascertaining incidence of severe hypoglycemia should be performed.

Even with this relatively low incidence of severe hypoglycemia, given the high prevalence of diabetes in the general population[1] and in the VA, there are likely tens of thousands of people in the US experiencing severe hypoglycemia every year. These episodes tend to be frightening, and may lead to more severe consequences (see Key Question #3 below) and to reluctance to pursue optimal blood sugar control.[140] They may also be associated with significant costs to the health care system.[141]

Key Question #2: What are the risk factors for severe hypoglycemia in adults with type 2 diabetes on one or more hypoglycemic agents (e.g., demographics, co-morbidities, diabetes treatment regimen, other medication use, goal and achieved HbA1c)?

We identified 14 articles from 12 studies that reported multivariate adjusted risk factor analyses for severe hypoglycemia in adults with type 2 diabetes on hypoglycemic mediations. Since these varied considerably with respect to risk factors evaluated (and their definitions), populations studied, and lengths of follow-up, the data were considered unsuitable for pooling. Transient causes (e.g., missed meal, excess exercise, alcohol use, acute infection) were not included.[142]

The factors evaluated in the 12 multivariate analyses are discussed below. In addition, genetic markers, marital status, smoking, alcohol consumption, polypharmacy, recent discharge from the hospital, congestive heart failure and use of ACE inhibitors were all identified in at least one of these 12 studies as independent risk factors for severe hypoglycemia. However, the findings for these risk factors were generally sparse, often conflicting, and ultimately inconclusive.

Independent Risk Factors

Factors most consistently and independently associated with risk include: intensive glycemic control (discussed above under Key Question #1), history of hypoglycemia, renal insufficiency, history of microvascular complications, longer diabetes duration, lower education level, African American race and history of dementia. History of hypoglycemia unawareness, gender, age and BMI are not consistently associated with risk, although higher age and lower BMI were associated with higher risk in the two largest studies.

Previous hypoglycemia which was evaluated in four studies, appears to be one of the strongest risk factors for a severe hypoglycemic event (three to nine-fold increased risk) and is often listed as a well known risk factor in reviews of this topic.[142, 143] Repeated episodes of hypoglycemia are thought to lead to autonomic insufficiency, a state in which patients become unaware of the common symptoms of low blood sugar, such as palpitations and lightheadedness. This unawareness may then lead to failure to take corrective action resulting in more episodes, thus establishing a vicious cycle.[144]

Renal insufficiency was evaluated in seven studies, five of which found it to be a significant independent risk factor for severe hypoglycemia. The two studies that did not find a significant association were either very small[102] or recorded very few episodes of severe hypoglycemia.[100] Renal insufficiency is a well known risk factor for hypoglycemia; the reduced clearance of insulin in the diseased kidney causes relative hyperinsulinemia which can lead to hypoglycemia.[141, 143] Hypoglycemia in renal insufficiency may also be due to reduced clearance of antidiabetic agents[145] and a decrease in renal gluconeogenesis.[146]

The relationship between renal insufficiency, hypoglycemic agents and incidence of severe hypoglycemia, however, is complicated. A nested case control study of 558 people with diabetes over the age of 65 on insulin, metformin or glyburide investigated whether renal function was an effect modifier for the association between glyburide or insulin use and hypoglycemia.[147] Since the study did not distinguish between severe and other forms of hypoglycemia, it was not included in our review. Results indicated that while renal function did not significantly modify risk of glyburide associated hypoglycemia, risk of insulin-associated hypoglycemia was, unexpectedly, attenuated by renal dysfunction.

The relationship between _non-renal microvascular disease_ and severe hypoglycemia was evaluated in five studies. In three of the five studies, there were significant positive associations between peripheral neuropathy (or its manifestation, leg ulcerations) and risk of severe hypoglycemia with risk ratios in the 1.2 to 2.4 range; the largest of these three studies, ACCORD,[3] found the lowest risk. In a fourth study, "history of microvascular disease," which also included renal disease, conferred a twofold increased risk of severe hypoglycemia (HR 2.1, 95% CI 1.5 to 3).[4] The pathophysiologic mechanism underlying this association is unclear. Although microvascular complications are an indicator of longstanding diabetes, duration of diabetes was often controlled for in these analyses.

Diabetes duration was associated with a modestly increased risk for severe hypoglycemia in studies (with odds ratios of less than 2) and is thought to be due to the compromised ability of people with advanced type 2 diabetes to mount an appropriate counter-regulatory hormonal (insulin, epinephrine, and glucagon) response to low blood sugar.[141, 143]

Demographic variables such as _African American race_ and _lower education level_ were both independently associated with a modestly increased risk of severe hypoglycemia. In the studies that evaluated race, blacks were significantly more likely than whites to experience severe hypoglycemia, with relative risks of 1.4 to 2.0. This association was independent of other known risk factors, such as education, that may track with race.[89]

Four of five studies that evaluated education, reported significant positive associations between lower education level and risk of severe hypoglycemia. One of these found the risk associated with low literacy rates, a more specific construct than education level, was associated with close to a four-fold increased risk. However this study was a case-control study that included fewer than 300 subjects leading to wide confidence intervals around the odds ratio.[104] It has been speculated that persons with low levels of education and literacy may not fully understand how to take their hypoglycemic medications or how to treat incipient hypoglycemia.

Dementia was found to be an independent risk factor for severe hypoglycemia in two of three studies. As is expected based on sample size, the much larger of these two studies (N=11,140)[4] found a modestly increased risk with a very tight confidence interval, whereas the smaller study (N=302),[92] found a larger risk with a very wide confidence interval. The only study that did not find an association was very small.[103] In addition, an article from ACCORD that was not included in our review because it was published in 2012, also found a significant association between poor cognitive function and risk of HMA.[148] Dementia may increase the likelihood of errors in self-medication and of inability to recognize and treat incipient hypoglycemia.[141]

Risk Factors NOT Found to be Independently Associated with Risk

Gender, age and low BMI were not consistently associated with risk, although age and low BMI were significantly predictive of risk of severe hypoglycemia in the two largest trials.[3, 4] It has been suggested that older people may be at increased risk due to diminished counter-regulatory and autonomic system responses to low blood sugar[149] and may be more likely to suffer from hypoglycemia unawareness.[150] Low BMI may contribute to hypoglycemia because of poor nutrition, decreased glucose absorption, or erratic meal plans. In contrast to age and BMI, the results for gender were conflicting in the two large trials: ACCORD found that women were at modestly increased risk compared with men whereas ADVANCE found no significant difference between men and women.

Impaired hypoglycemic awareness was only evaluated in one of our included studies.[84] Although this study found a significant increased risk, it employed a weak study design (cross sectional) and had relatively few subjects (N=401).

Other Literature

We did not identify any other systematic reviews that evaluated risk factors for severe hypoglycemia in people with type 2 diabetes. One literature survey included six prospective and five retrospective studies that enrolled at least 50 participants all on insulin followed for at least 6 months.[151] The risk factors identified included impaired hypoglycemia awareness, advanced age, longer duration of diabetes and of insulin therapy. HbA1c at baseline and dose of insulin were not found to increase risk. However this study included only insulin treated patients, did not limit its review to studies using multivariate analysis, and antedated publication of the three large trials of intensive versus conventional control.

An unpublished abstract examining VA administrative data reported the following risk factors for an inpatient or outpatient diagnosis of hypoglycemia: prior hypoglycemia, history of ketoacidosis or hyperosmolar coma, high HbA1c levels, recent initiation of a new medication, recent hospitalization, use of secretagogues, insulin, fluoroquinolones or tricyclic antidepressants, higher age, low SES (which often correlates with education level) and unmarried status. It is unclear from the abstract how the diagnoses were confirmed and what the severity of the episodes were. In addition, a paper published after our literature search was concluded indicated that dementia and cognitive impairment were independent risk factors for hypoglycemia among older veterans,[139] consistent with our findings.

Limitations of Available Studies

The data are relatively sparse and almost certainly reflect publication bias (negative analyses are less likely to be published). In addition we were unable to pool results across studies due to the heterogeneity of the study designs, analytical methods, and risk factors assessed. Finally, only two studies used negative binomial or zero inflated poisson[16, 84, 93] methodology which may be less likely than standard regression techniques to yield spurious associations in situations in which there are frequent zero counts.[152]

Conclusion for Key Question #2

Independent risk factors for severe hypoglycemia in persons with type 2 diabetes on hypoglycemic medication include: intensive diabetes control, history of hypoglycemia, renal insufficiency, history of microvascular complications, longer diabetes duration, lower education level, African American race and history of dementia. Gender, age and BMI are not consistently associated with risk, although in the two largest studies, higher age and lower BMI were significantly associated with higher risk.

Key Question #3. What is the effect of severe hypoglycemia on other outcomes in adults with type 2 diabetes on one or more hypoglycemic agents (e.g., quality of life, mortality, morbidity, utilization)?

Severe hypoglycemia causes brain fuel deprivation that, if uncorrected, can lead to neurological compromise and death.[143] There is uncertainty about a possible link between hypoglycemia and mortality, cardiovascular events, and other adverse health outcomes.[153-155] Based on studies included in this review, we found no evidence of increased short-term mortality and limited evidence that a history of severe hypoglycemia increases long-term mortality. Few cardiovascular events were reported; coma and seizures were present in 5% to 71% of patients with severe hypoglycemia.

A recent study of over 850,000 patients found greater odds of an acute cardiovascular event during a one year period in type 2 diabetic patients who also experienced a hypoglycemic event (not necessarily severe) during that period (OR 1.79, 95% CI 1.69 to 1.89). The analysis included adjustment for baseline cardiovascular risk factors, comorbidities, and prior cardiovascular events (all of which were significantly more prevalent in the hypoglycemia group).[156] In a study of adverse events reported to the Food and Drug Administration from 1998 through 2005, there were 9597 reports of insulin-associated disability or other serious but non-fatal outcome.[157] However, in a study of patients hospitalized with acute MI, not all of whom had diabetes, spontaneous hypoglycemia in patients not treated with insulin was associated with increased risk for mortality; among patients treated with insulin, hypoglycemia was not associated with increased risk for mortality. This would suggest that hypoglycemia, itself, does not cause adverse events but is, instead, a marker of severe illness.[158] People who are likely to experience hypoglycemia may also be likely to experience other serious health outcomes due to other risk factors.[155]

It is well known that cognitive and psychomotor function decline during a hypoglycemic episode.[159, 160] Therefore, it is theorized that driving performance would be affected. However, whether severe hypoglycemia is associated with an increase in motor vehicle crashes is uncertain. Data from early studies are of questionable value as a result of improvements in methods for self-monitoring of blood glucose and changes in available medications.[161] A more recent study found a nearly four-fold increased risk of a history of severe hypoglycemia in those who experienced a motor vehicle crash.[129]

Much of the information about driving performance is from laboratory studies where hypoglycemia is induced and driving simulators are used. In a recent study of 20 type 2 diabetic individuals with normal hypoglycemic awareness (mean age 52 years, all of whom had a driver's license for at least 2 years), 11 of the 20 felt hypoglycemic. Of those 11, five (45%) said they would measure their blood glucose and six (55%) said they would not drive. Nine of the 20 "maybe" felt hypoglycemic. Of those nine, three (33%) said they would drive, two (22%) said they would "maybe" drive, two (22%) said they would measure their glucose and two (22%) said they would not drive.[130] It is unknown how results from studies of this type translate to actual driving performance or behavior.

Long-term effects of hypoglycemia, especially repeated episodes of severe hypoglycemia, on cognitive performance are not fully understood.[159, 160] Results, to date, in patients with type 2 diabetes have been mixed.[92, 94] The DCCT/EDIC trial in patients with type 1 diabetes found neither frequency of severe hypoglycemia nor initial treatment group assignment (intensive versus conventional therapy) were associated with cognitive decline over 18 years based on a battery of 17 tests representing eight cognitive domains.[162] The ACCORD-MIND study reported no differences in cognitive outcomes between intensive treatment and standard treatment groups at 40 months. The authors did not relate their findings to the presence or absence of severe hypoglycemic episodes.[163]

Data from the Edinburgh Type 2 Diabetes Study were recently published.[164] Participants, all age 60 to75 years, were asked about severe hypoglycemic events. A history of severe hypoglycemia (one or more episodes) was associated with lower cognitive ability as reflected by the Letter-Number Sequencing test (p=0.03), the Trail-Making Test (p=0.004), and a composite score based on seven cognitive tests (p=0.04). Results were adjusted for prior cognitive ability, demographic characteristics and comorbid conditions. Similar findings were noted for the analysis based on severe hypoglycemia in the year preceding cognitive testing.

Potential reasons for differences across studies have been suggested in the literature. Many studies of cognitive function completed to date may not have sufficient follow-up time to adequately address long-term effects.[159] Differences observed between studies may be due to differential effects of hypoglycemia on the brain in younger versus older people.[160] Increased risk of dementia associated with type 2 diabetes may be due to other factors (e.g., depression, vascular disease, comorbid conditions and associated medications and genetic predisposition).[165] Alternatively, an observed association between hypoglycemia and cognitive decline may be due to the fact that patients with cognitive decline may be less able to manage their diabetes and therefore may experience more hypoglycemic events.[159]

Hypoglycemia, particularly severe hypoglycemia, results in utilization of health care resources. In studies included in this review, we observed that between 0% and 31% of episodes of severe hypoglycemia were seen in an emergency department and between 0% and 33% of episodes resulted in hospital admission. Increased physician visits were also reported. A recent systematic review recommended increased hospitalization and primary care visits for post-hypoglycemic patients.[166] Citing the potential for repeat hypoglycemia, as reported in studies of post-hypoglycemic type 2 diabetes patients taking oral hypoglycemic agents and first treated for a hypoglycemic episode in a prehospital environment, the authors recommended conservative management (i.e., transportation of all patients to a hospital for observation and treatment). They also encouraged the development of evidence-based interventions to increase primary or specialty care visits by post-hypoglycemic patients.

In a study examining nationally representative data, Budnitz et al.[167] estimated that insulin, metformin, glyburide and glipizide were implicated in 13%, 2.3%, 2.2%, and 1.5% of all emergency department visits in the United States in persons age 65 and older. These four were among the top 10 most commonly implicated medications.[167] In a more recent study, this group estimated that insulin and oral hypoglycemic agents accounted for 25% of all adverse drug event-associated emergency hospitalizations in the United States in 2007-2009.[168] These studies did not link the emergency department visits or hospitalizations to episodes of severe hypoglycemia.

Limitations of Available Studies

Few studies that address outcomes of severe hypoglycemic episodes include appropriate control groups. In addition, many outcomes of interest were not widely reported.

Conclusion for Key Question #3

There is good data that severe hypoglycemia is associated with an increased risk of the following outcomes: all-cause mortality (particularly long-term), neurological events (other than non-fatal stroke), hospital and emergency department utilization, and decreased quality of life. There is limited data about many other outcomes of interest including non-fatal MI, non-fatal stroke, cognitive decline, motor vehicle accidents, falls and traumatic injuries, work productivity, and other medical service utilization. In the absence of appropriate control groups it is unclear if many of these outcomes are hypoglycemia-related or simply reflect the age and co-morbidity burden of the population.

RECOMMENDATIONS FOR FUTURE RESEARCH

Key Question #1: Larger population-based prospective studies of people on a variety of hypoglycemic agents that employ accurate methods for ascertaining incidence of severe hypoglycemia should be performed. Studies need to control for or stratify outcomes by important patient, disease and comorbidity factors including: age, gender, race/ethnicity, socio-economic and marital status, disease duration and severity (e.g., HbA1c level, presence or absence of diabetic complications).

Key Question #2: Future research should include studies in VA patients and include the more intriguing possible risk factors including smoking or recent hospital discharge. In addition, future research may lead to the development of a risk factor index if outcomes are significant enough to warrant risk stratification.

Key Question #3: Future studies of outcomes associated with severe hypoglycemia should be prospective, use a uniform and generally accepted definition of severe hypoglycemia, and include, as controls, people with medication-treated diabetes who have not experienced severe hypoglycemia. Also, studies should clearly distinguish between short-term or episode-related versus long-term consequences.

Specific future research needs include:

a. To clarify the association between hypoglycemia and cardiovascular events, research is needed to better understand the effects of hypoglycemia on blood constituents and the vascular system and larger clinical trials are needed to determine whether hypoglycemia is a cause of cardiovascular events.[153, 154] Better understanding of the role of hypoglycemia in patients already at risk for developing vascular disease is also needed.[153]

b. There is a need for a large-scale, prospective study of accident rates in patients with diabetes compared to appropriate control groups.[161] Better understanding is needed of which driving skills are most likely to be affected by hypoglycemia, at what level of blood glucose driving impairments become observable, and whether results obtained in a laboratory translate to road conditions.[134]

c. Additional research is needed to assess the overall effect of hypoglycemia on patients with type 2 diabetes including quality of life outcomes (both work and recreational). To date, much of the research has focused on type 1 diabetes and the emphasis has been on hypoglycemia as a safety issue.[169]

d. To assess the effect of hypoglycemia on cognitive function, large-scale epidemiological studies with detailed phenotyping of clinical variables and randomized trials of interventions (therapeutic and preventive) that include cognitive testing and brain structure/function assessments are needed.[165, 170]

REFERENCES

1.   Danaei G, Finucane MM, Lu Y, et al. National, regional, and global trends in fasting plasma glucose and diabetes prevalence since 1980: systematic analysis of health examination surveys and epidemiological studies with 370 country-years and 2.7 million participants. *Lancet.* 2011;378(9785):31-40.

2.   Miller DR, Safford MM, Pogach LM. Who has diabetes? Best estimates of diabetes prevalence in the Department of Veterans Affairs based on computerized patient data. *Diabetes Care.* 2004;27 Suppl 2:B10-21.

3.   Action to Control Cardiovascular Risk in Diabetes Study G, Gerstein HC, Miller ME, et al. Effects of intensive glucose lowering in type 2 diabetes. *N Engl J Med.* 2008;358(24):2545-2559.

4.   Advance, Patel A, MacMahon S, et al. Intensive blood glucose control and vascular outcomes in patients with type 2 diabetes. *N Engl J Med.* 2008;358(24):2560-2572.

5.   Duckworth W, Abraira C, Moritz T, et al. Glucose control and vascular complications in veterans with type 2 diabetes. *N Engl J Med.* 2009;360(2):129-139.

6.   Ismail-Beigi F, Craven T, Banerji MA, et al. Effect of intensive treatment of hyperglycaemia on microvascular outcomes in type 2 diabetes: an analysis of the ACCORD randomised trial. *Lancet.* 2010;376(9739):419-430.

7.   Action to Control Cardiovascular Risk in Diabetes Study G, Gerstein HC, Miller ME, et al. Long-term effects of intensive glucose lowering on cardiovascular outcomes. *N Engl J Med.* 2011;364(9):818-828.

8.   Kelly TN, Bazzano LA, Fonseca VA, Thethi TK, Reynolds K, He J. Systematic review: glucose control and cardiovascular disease in type 2 diabetes. *Ann Intern Med.* 2009;151(6):394-403.

9.   Hemmingsen B, Lund SS, Gluud C, et al. Targeting intensive glycaemic control versus targeting conventional glycaemic control for type 2 diabetes mellitus. *Cochrane Database Syst Rev.* 2011(6):CD008143.

10. Ray KK, Seshasai SR, Wijesuriya S, et al. Effect of intensive control of glucose on cardiovascular outcomes and death in patients with diabetes mellitus: a meta-analysis of randomised controlled trials. *Lancet.* 2009;373(9677):1765-1772.

11. Boussageon R, Bejan-Angoulvant T, Saadatian-Elahi M, et al. Effect of intensive glucose lowering treatment on all cause mortality, cardiovascular death, and microvascular events in type 2 diabetes: meta-analysis of randomised controlled trials. *BMJ.* 2011;343:d4169.

12. Pogach L, Aron D. Balancing hypoglycemia and glycemic control: a public health approach for insulin safety. *JAMA.* 2010;303(20):2076-2077.

13.   Higgins JP, Green, S., eds. Cochrane Handbook for Systematic Reviews of Interventions
      Version 5.1.0 (Updated March 2011). In: Higgins JP, Green, S., ed. Vol 5.1.0: The
      Cochrane Collaboration; 2011: http://www.cochrane-handbook.org. Accessed August 29,
      2011.

14.   Schulz KF, Grimes DA. Allocation concealment in randomised trials: defending against
      deciphering. *Lancet.* 2002;359(9306):614-618.

15.   Berntorp K, Haglund M, Larsen S, Petruckevitch A, Landin-Olsson M, Swedish BSG.
      Initiation of biphasic insulin aspart 30/70 in subjects with type 2 diabetes mellitus in a
      largely primary care-based setting in Sweden. *Primary care diabetes.* 2011;5(2):89-94.

16.   Davis TME, Brown SGA, Jacobs IG, Bulsara M, Bruce DG, Davis WA. Determinants of
      severe hypoglycemia complicating type 2 diabetes: the Fremantle diabetes study. *J Clin
      Endocrinol Metab.* 2010;95(5):2240-2247.

17.   Holstein A, Plaschke A, Egberts EH. Lower incidence of severe hypoglycaemia in
      patients with type 2 diabetes treated with glimepiride versus glibenclamide. *Diabetes-
      Metab Res.* 2001;17(6):467-473.

18.   Marre M, Pinget M, Gin H, et al. Insulin detemir improves glycaemic control with less
      hypoglycaemia and no weight gain: 52-week data from the PREDICTIVE study in a
      cohort of French patients with type 1 or type 2 diabetes. *Diabetes Metab.* 2009;35(6):469-
      475.

19.   Murata GH, Duckworth WC, Shah JH, Wendel CS, Mohler MJ, Hoffman RM.
      Hypoglycemia in stable, insulin-treated veterans with type 2 diabetes: a prospective study
      of 1662 episodes. *J Diabetes Complicat.* 2005;19(1):10-17.

20.   Pencek R, Roddy T, Peters Y, et al. Safety of pramlintide added to mealtime insulin in
      patients with type 1 or type 2 diabetes: a large observational study. *Diabetes Obes Metab.*
      2010;12:548-551.

21.   UK Prospective Diabetes Study Group U. Intensive blood-glucose control with
      sulphonylureas or insulin compared with conventional treatment and risk of
      complications in patients with type 2 diabetes. *Lancet.* 1998;352:837-853.

22.   Valensi P, Benroubi M, Borzi V, et al. Initiating insulin therapy with, or switching
      existing insulin therapy to, biphasic insulin aspart 30/70 (NovoMix 30) in routine care:
      safety and effectiveness in patients with type 2 diabetes in the IMPROVE observational
      study. *Int J Clin Pract.* 2009;63(3):522-531.

23.   Asche CV, McAdam-Marx C, Shane-McWhorter L, Sheng X, Plauschinat CA.
      Evaluation of adverse events of oral antihyperglycemic monotherapy experienced by a
      geriatric population in a real-world setting: a retrospective cohort analysis. *Drugs Aging.*
      2008;25(7):611-622.

24.   Bodmer M, Meier C, Kr, et al. Metformin, sulfonylureas, or other antidiabetes drugs and the risk of lactic acidosis or hypoglycemia: a nested case-control analysis. *Diabetes Care.* 2008;31(11):2086-2091.

25.   Leese GP, Wang J, Broomhall J, et al. Frequency of severe hypoglycemia requiring emergency treatment in type 1 and type 2 diabetes: a population-based study of health service resource use. *Diabetes Care.* 2003;26(4):1176-1180.

26.   Nichols GA, Gandra SR, Chiou C-F, Anthony MS, Alexander-Bridges M, Brown JB. Successes and challenges of insulin therapy for type 2 diabetes in a managed-care setting. *Curr Med Res Opin.* 2010;26(1):9-15.

27.   Quilliam BJ, Simeone JC, Ozbay AB. Risk Factors for Hypoglycemia-Related Hospitalization in Patients with Type 2 Diabetes: A Nested Case-Control Study. *Clin Ther.* 2011.

28.   Stahl M, Berger W. Higher incidence of severe hypoglycaemia leading to hospital admission in Type 2 diabetic patients treated with long-acting versus short-acting sulphonylureas. *Diabetic Med.* 1999;16(7):586-590.

29.   UK Prospective Diabetes Study Group. Effect of intensive blood-glucose control with metformin on complications in overweight patients with type 2 diabetes (UKPDS 34). *The Lancet.* 1998;352(9131):854-865.

30.   Abraira C, Colwell JA, Nuttall FQ, et al. Veterans Affairs Cooperative Study on glycemic control and complications in type II diabetes (VA CSDM). Results of the feasibility trial. Veterans Affairs Cooperative Study in Type II Diabetes. *Diabetes Care.* 1995;18(8):1113-1123.

31.   Raskin P, Gylvin T, Weng W, Chaykin L. Comparison of insulin detemir and insulin glargine using a basal-bolus regimen in a randomized, controlled clinical study in patients with type 2 diabetes. *Diabetes-Metab Res.* 2009;25(6):542-548.

32.   Drouin P, Standl E, Group tDMS. Gliclazide modified release: results of a 2-year study of patients with type 2 diabetes. *Diabetes Obes Metab.* 2004;6:414-421.

33.   Haak T, Tiengo A, Draeger E, Suntum M, Waldhausl W. Lower within-subject variability of fasting blood glucose and reduced weight gain with insulin detemir compared to NPH insulin in patients with type 2 diabetes. *Diabetes Obes Metab.* 2005;7(1):56-64.

34.   Ratner RE, Want LL, Fineman MS, et al. Adjunctive therapy with the amylin analogue pramlintide leads to a combined improvement in glycemic and weight control in insulin-treated subjects with type 2 diabetes. *Diabetes Technol The* 2002;4(1):51-61.

35.   Rosenstock J, Fonseca V, McGill JB, et al. Similar progression of diabetic retinopathy with insulin glargine and neutral protamine Hagedorn (NPH) insulin in patients with type 2 diabetes: a long-term, randomised, open-label study. *Diabetologia.* 2009;52(9):1778-1788.

36.   Buse JB, Wolffenbuttel BHR, Herman WH, et al. The DURAbility of Basal versus Lispro mix 75/25 insulin Efficacy (DURABLE) trial: comparing the durability of lispro mix 75/25 and glargine. *Diabetes Care.* 2011;34(2):249-255.

37.   Kennedy L, Herman WH, Strange P, Harris A, Team GA. Impact of active versus usual algorithmic titration of basal insulin and point-of-care versus laboratory measurement of HbA1c on glycemic control in patients with type 2 diabetes: the Glycemic Optimization with Algorithms and Labs at Point of Care (GOAL A1C) trial. *Diabetes Care.* 2006;29(1):1-8.

38.   Davies M, Storms F, Shutler S, Bianchi-Biscay M, Gomis R, Group AS. Improvement of glycemic control in subjects with poorly controlled type 2 diabetes: comparison of two treatment algorithms using insulin glargine. *Diabetes Care.* 2005;28(6):1282-1288.

39.   Rosenstock J, Schwartz SL, Clark CM, Jr., Park GD, Donley DW, Edwards MB. Basal insulin therapy in type 2 diabetes: 28-week comparison of insulin glargine (HOE 901) and NPH insulin. *Diabetes Care.* 2001;24(4):631-636.

40.   Rosenstock J, Davies M, Home PD, Larsen J, Koenen C, Schernthaner G. A randomised, 52-week, treat-to-target trial comparing insulin detemir with insulin glargine when administered as add-on to glucose-lowering drugs in insulin-naive people with type 2 diabetes. *Diabetologia.* 2008;51(3):408-416.

41.   Riddle MC, Rosenstock J, Gerich J, Insulin Glargine Study I. The treat-to-target trial: randomized addition of glargine or human NPH insulin to oral therapy of type 2 diabetic patients. *Diabetes Care.* 2003;26(11):3080-3086.

42.   Heine RJ, Van Gaal LF, Johns D, et al. Exenatide versus insulin glargine in patients with suboptimally controlled type 2 diabetes: a randomized trial. *Ann Intern Med.* 2005;143(8):559-569.

43.   Holman RR, Farmer AJ, Davies MJ, et al. Three-year efficacy of complex insulin regimens in type 2 diabetes. *N Engl J Med.* 2009;361(18):1736-1747.

44.   Fritsche A, Schweitzer MA, x00E, ring H-U, Study G. Glimepiride combined with morning insulin glargine, bedtime neutral protamine hagedorn insulin, or bedtime insulin glargine in patients with type 2 diabetes. A randomized, controlled trial. *Ann Intern Med.* 2003;138(12):952-959.

45.   Rayman G, Profozic V, Middle M. Insulin glulisine imparts effective glycaemic control in patients with Type 2 diabetes. *Diabetes Res Clin Pr.* 2006;76:304-312.

46.   Dailey GE, 3rd, Noor MA, Park J-S, Bruce S, Fiedorek FT. Glycemic control with glyburide/metformin tablets in combination with rosiglitazone in patients with type 2 diabetes: a randomized, double-blind trial. *Am J Med.* 2004;116(4):223-229.

47.   Anderson JH, Jr., Brunelle RL, Keohane P, et al. Mealtime treatment with insulin analog improves postprandial hyperglycemia and hypoglycemia in patients with non-insulin-dependent diabetes mellitus. Multicenter Insulin Lispro Study Group. *Arch Int Med.* 1997;157(11):1249-1255.

48.   Liebl A, Prager R, Binz K, et al. Comparison of insulin analogue regimens in people with type 2 diabetes mellitus in the PREFER study: a randomized controlled trial. *Diabetes Obes Metab.* 2009;11:45-52.

49.   Matthews DR, Dejager S, Ahren B, et al. Vildagliptin add-on to metformin produces similar efficacy and reduced hypoglycaemic risk compared with glimepiride, with no weight gain: results from a 2-year study. *Diabetes Obes Metab.* 2010;12(9):780-789.

50.   Seck T, Nauck M, Sheng D, et al. Safety and efficacy of treatment with sitagliptin or glipizide in patients with type 2 diabetes inadequately controlled on metformin: a 2-year study. *Int J Clin Pract.* 2010;64(5):562-576.

51.   Garber A, Henry RR, Ratner R, et al. Liraglutide, a once-daily human glucagon-like peptide 1 analogue, provides sustained improvements in glycaemic control and weight for 2 years as monotherapy compared with glimepiride in patients with type 2 diabetes. *Diabetes Obes Metab.* 2011;13(4):348-356.

52.   Arechavaleta R, Seck T, Chen Y, et al. Efficacy and safety of treatment with sitagliptin or glimepiride in patients with type 2 diabetes inadequately controlled on metformin monotherapy: a randomized, double-blind, non-inferiority trial. *Diabetes Obes Metab.* 2011;13(2):160-168.

53.   Nauck M, Frid A, Hermansen K, et al. Efficacy and safety comparison of liraglutide, glimepiride, and placebo, all in combination with metformin, in type 2 diabetes: the LEAD (liraglutide effect and action in diabetes)-2 study. *Diabetes Care.* 2009;32(1):84-90.

54.   Russell-Jones D, Vaag A, Schmitz O, et al. Liraglutide vs insulin glargine and placebo in combination with metformin and sulfonylurea therapy in type 2 diabetes mellitus (LEAD-5 met+SU): a randomised controlled trial. *Diabetologia.* 2009;52(10):2046-2055.

55.   Chou HS, Palmer JP, Jones AR, et al. Initial treatment with fixed-dose combination rosiglitazone/glimepiride in patients with previously untreated type 2 diabetes. *Diabetes Obes Metab.* 2008;10(8):626-637.

56.   Kendall DM, Riddle MC, Rosenstock J, et al. Effects of exenatide (exendin-4) on glycemic control over 30 weeks in patients with type 2 diabetes treated with metformin and a sulfonylurea. *Diabetes Care.* 2005;28(5):1083-1091.

57.   Schernthaner G, Grimaldi A, Di Mario U, et al. GUIDE study: double-blind comparison of once-daily gliclazide MR and glimepiride in type 2 diabetic patients. *Eur J Clin Invest.* 2004;34(8):535-542.

58. Bari2D, Frye RL, August P, et al. A randomized trial of therapies for type 2 diabetes and coronary artery disease. *N Engl J Med.* 2009;360(24):2503-2515.

59. Saloranta C, Hershon K, Ball M, Dickinson S, Holmes D. Efficacy and safety of nateglinide in type 2 diabetic patients with modest fasting hyperglycemia. *J Clin Endocrinol Metab.* 2002;87(9):4171-4176.

60. Aschner P, Katzeff HL, Guo H, et al. Efficacy and safety of monotherapy of sitagliptin compared with metformin in patients with type 2 diabetes. *Diabetes Obes Metab.* 2010;12(3):252-261.

61. Bonds DE, Miller ME, Bergenstal RM, et al. The association between symptomatic, severe hypoglycaemia and mortality in type 2 diabetes: retrospective epidemiological analysis of the ACCORD study. *BMJ.* 2010;340:b4909.

62. Waugh N, Cummins E, Royle P, et al. Newer agents for blood glucose control in type 2 diabetes: systematic review and economic evaluation. *Health Technol Assess.* 2010;14(36):1-248.

63. Shyangdan DS, Royle P, Clar C, Sharma P, Waugh N, Snaith A. Glucagon-like peptide analogues for type 2 diabetes mellitus. *Cochrane Database Syst Rev.* 2011(10):CD006423.

64. Richter B, Bandeira-Echtler E, Bergerhoff K, Lerch CL. Dipeptidyl peptidase-4 (DPP-4) inhibitors for type 2 diabetes mellitus. *Cochrane Database Syst Rev.* 2008(2):CD006739.

65. Swinnen SG, Simon AC, Holleman F, Hoekstra JB, Devries JH. Insulin detemir versus insulin glargine for type 2 diabetes mellitus. *Cochrane Database Syst Rev.* 2011(7):CD006383.

66. Horvath K, Jeitler K, Berghold A, et al. Long-acting insulin analogues versus NPH insulin (human isophane insulin) for type 2 diabetes mellitus. *Cochrane Database Syst Rev.* 2007(2):CD005613.

67. Siebenhofer A, Plank J, Berghold A, et al. Short acting insulin analogues versus regular human insulin in patients with diabetes mellitus. *Cochrane Database Syst Rev.* 2006(2):CD003287.

68. Tran K BS, Li H, Cimon K, Daneman D, Simpson SH, Campbell K. *Long-active insulin analogues for diabetes mellitus: meta-analysis of clinical outcomes and assessment of costeffectiveness* [Technoogy Report no 87]. Ottawa: Canadian Agency for Drugs and Technologies in Health; 2007.

69. Goudswaard AN, Furlong NJ, Rutten GE, Stolk RP, Valk GD. Insulin monotherapy versus combinations of insulin with oral hypoglycaemic agents in patients with type 2 diabetes mellitus. *Cochrane Database Syst Rev.* 2004(4):CD003418.

70. Clar C, Royle P, Waugh N. Adding pioglitazone to insulin containing regimens in type 2 diabetes: systematic review and meta-analysis. *PLoS One.* 2009;4(7):e6112.

71.   Black C, Donnelly P, McIntyre L, Royle PL, Shepherd JP, Thomas S. Meglitinide analogues for type 2 diabetes mellitus. *Cochrane Database Syst Rev.* 2007(2):CD004654.

72.   Donnelly LA, Morris AD, Frier BM, et al. Frequency and predictors of hypoglycaemia in Type 1 and insulin-treated Type 2 diabetes: a population-based study. *Diabetic Med.* 2005;22(6):749-755.

73.   Chan S-P, Ji L-N, Nitiyanant W, Baik SH, Sheu WHH. Hypoglycemic symptoms in patients with type 2 diabetes in Asia-Pacific-Real-life effectiveness and care patterns of diabetes management: the RECAP-DM study. *Diabetes Res Clin Pr.* 2010;89(2):e30-32.

74.   Neil BJ, Baines A, Clothier B, Nelson DB, Bloomfield HE. Self-Monitoring of Blood Glucose in Diabetic Patients Not Taking Insulin: Does It Affect Hypoglycemia? *Federal Practitioner.* 2007 2007:27-33.

75.   Moen MF, Zhan M, Hsu VD, et al. Frequency of Hypoglycemia and Its Significance in Chronic Kidney Disease. *Clin J Am Soc Nephrol.* 2009;4:1121-1127.

76.   Henderson JN, Allen KV, Deary IJ, Frier BM. Hypoglycaemia in insulin-treated Type 2 diabetes: frequency, symptoms and impaired awareness. *Diabetic Med.* 2003;20(12):1016-1021.

77.   Honkasalo M, Elonheimo O, Sane T. Many diabetic patients with recurrent severe hypoglycemias hold a valid driving license. A community-based study in insulin-treated patients with diabetes. *Traffic Injury Prevention.* 2010;11(3):258-262.

78.   Sarkar U, Karter AJ, Liu JY, Moffet HH, Adler NE, Schillinger D. Hypoglycemia is more common among type 2 diabetes patients with limited health literacy: the Diabetes Study of Northern California (DISTANCE). *J Gen Inern Med.* 2010;25(9):962-968.

79.   Lecomte P, Romon I, Fosse S, Simon D, Fagot-Campagna A. Self-monitoring of blood glucose in people with type 1 and type 2 diabetes living in France: the Entred study 2001. *Diabetes Metab.* 2008;34(3):219-226.

80.   Jennings AM, Wilson RM, Ward JD. Symptomatic hypoglycemia in NIDDM patients treated with oral hypoglycemic agents. *Diabetes Care.* 1989;12(3):203-208.

81.   Marrett E, Stargardt T, Mavros P, Alexander CM. Patient-reported outcomes in a survey of patients treated with oral antihyperglycaemic medications: associations with hypoglycaemia and weight gain. *Diabetes Obes Metab.* 2009;11(12):1138-1144.

82.   Pettersson B, Rosenqvist U, Deleskog A, Journath G, Wandell P. Self-reported experience of hypoglycemia among adults with type 2 diabetes mellitus (Exhype). *Diabetes Res Clin Pr.* 2011;92(1):19-25.

83.   Stargardt T, Gonder-Frederick L, Krobot KJ, Alexander CM. Fear of hypoglycaemia: defining a minimum clinically important difference in patients with type 2 diabetes. *Health Qual Life Out.* 2009;7:91.

84. Akram K, Pedersen-Bjergaard U, Carstensen B, Borch-Johnsen K, Thorsteinsson B. Frequency and risk factors of severe hypoglycaemia in insulin-treated Type 2 diabetes: a cross-sectional survey. *Diabetic Med.* 2006;23(7):750-756.

85. Alvarez Guisasola F, et al. Hypoglycaemic symptoms, treatment satisfaction, adherence and their associations with glycaemic goal in patients with type 2 diabetes mellitus: findings from the Real-Life Effectiveness and Care Patterns of Diabetes Management (RECAP-DM) Study. *Diabetes Obes Metab.* 2008;10 Suppl 1:25-32.

86. Williams SA, Pollack MF, Dibonaventura M. Effects of hypoglycemia on health-related quality of life, treatment satisfaction and healthcare resource utilization in patients with type 2 diabetes mellitus. *Diabetes Res Clin Pr.* 2011;91(3):363-370.

87. Marrett E, Radican L, Davies MJ, Zhang Q. Assessment of severity and frequency of self-reported hypoglycemia on quality of life in patients with type 2 diabetes treated with oral antihyperglycemic agents: A survey study. *BMC Research Notes.* 2011;4(251).

88. Lee LJ, Yu AP, Johnson SJ, et al. Direct costs associated with initiating NPH insulin versus glargine in patients with type 2 diabetes: a retrospective database analysis. *Diabetes Res Clin Pr.* 2010;87(1):108-116.

89. Miller ME, Bonds DE, Gerstein HC, et al. The effects of baseline characteristics, glycaemia treatment approach, and glycated haemoglobin concentration on the risk of severe hypoglycaemia: post hoc epidemiological analysis of the ACCORD study. *BMJ.* 2010;340-4.

90. Zoungas S, Patel A, Chalmers J, et al. Severe hypoglycemia and risks of vascular events and death. *N Engl J Med.* 2010;363(15):1410-1418.

91. Stratton I MS, Holman R, Turner R. Hypertenstion in Diabetes Study IV. Therapeutic requirements to maintain tight blood pressure control. *Diabetologia.* 1996;39:1554-1561.

92. Bruce DG, Davis WA, Casey GP, et al. Severe hypoglycaemia and cognitive impairment in older patients with diabetes: the Fremantle Diabetes Study. *Diabetologia.* 2009;52(9):1808-1815.

93. Davis WA, Brown SGA, Jacobs IG, et al. Angiotensin-converting enzyme insertion/ deletion polymorphism and severe hypoglycemia complicating type 2 diabetes: the Fremantle Diabetes Study. *J Clin Endocrinol Metab.* 2011;96(4):E696-700.

94. Whitmer RA, Karter AJ, Yaffe K, Quesenberry CP, Jr., Selby JV. Hypoglycemic episodes and risk of dementia in older patients with type 2 diabetes mellitus. *JAMA.* 2009;301(15):1565-1572.

95. Fadini GP, Rigato M, Tiengo A, Avogaro A. Characteristics and mortality of type 2 diabetic patients hospitalized for severe iatrogenic hypoglycemia. *Diabetes Res Clin Pr.* 2009;84(3):267-272.

96.   Sugarman JR. Hypoglycemia associated hospitalizations in a population with a high prevalence of non-insulin-dependent diabetes mellitus. *Diabetes Res Clin Pr.* 1991;14(2):139-147.

97.   Shorr RI, Ray WA, Daugherty JR, Griffin MR. Incidence and Risk Factors for Serious Hypoglycemia in Older Persons Using Insulin or Sulfonylureas. *Arch Intern Med.* 1997;157:1681-1686.

98.   Stepka M, Rogala H, Czyzyk A. Hypoglycemia: a major problem in the management of diabetes in the elderly. *Aging-Clin Exp Res.* 1993;5(2):117-121.

99.   Hepburn DA, MacLeod KM, Pell AC, Scougal IJ, Frier BM. Frequency and symptoms of hypoglycaemia experienced by patients with type 2 diabetes treated with insulin. *Diabetic Med.* 1993;10(3):231-237.

100. Miller CD, Phillips LS, Ziemer DC, Gallina DL, Cook CB, El-Kebbi IM. Hypoglycemia in patients with type 2 diabetes mellitus. *Arch Int Med.* 2001;161(13):1653-1659.

101. Shen JJ, Washington EL. Identification of diabetic complications among minority populations. *Ethnic Dis.* 2008;18(2):136-140.

102. Holstein A, Hahn M, Stumvoll M, Kovacs P. The E23K variant of KCNJ11 and the risk for severe sulfonylurea-induced hypoglycemia in patients with type 2 diabetes. *Hormone Metab Res.* 2009;41(5):387-390.

103. Holstein A, Hahn M, Patzer O, Seeringer A, Kovacs P, Stingl J. Impact of clinical factors and CYP2C9 variants for the risk of severe sulfonylurea-induced hypoglycemia. *Eur J Clin Pharmacol.* 2011;67(5):471-476.

104. Duran-Nah JJ, Rodriguez-Morales A, Smitheram J, Correa-Medina C. Risk factors associated with sympotmatic hyopglycemia in type 2 diabetes mellitus patients. *Revista de Investigacion.* 2008;60(6):451-458.

105. Asplund K, Wiholm BE, Lundman B. Severe hypoglycaemia during treatment with glipizide. *Diabetic Med.* 1991;8(8):726-731.

106. Sato H, Lattermann R, Carvalho G, et al. Perioperative glucose and insulin administration while maintaining normoglycemia (GIN therapy) in patients undergoing major liver resection. *Anes Analg.* 2010;110(6):1711-1718.

107. Holstein A, Plaschke A, Hammer C, Egberts EH. Characteristics and time course of severe glimepiride- versus glibenclamide-induced hypoglycaemia. *Eur J Clin Pharmacol.* 2003;59(2):91-97.

108. Sotiropoulos A, Skliros EA, Tountas C, Apostolou U, Peppas TA, Pappas SI. Risk factors for severe hypoglycaemia in type 2 diabetic patients admitted to hospital in Piraeus, Greece. *Eastern Mediterranean Health Journal.* 2005;11(3):485-489.

109. Holstein A, Plaschke A, Egberts EH. Clinical characterisation of severe hypoglycaemia—a prospective population-based study. *Exp Clin Endocr Diab.* 2003;111(6):364-369.

110. Buse JB, Wolffenbuttel BHR, Herman WH, et al. DURAbility of basal versus lispro mix 75/25 insulin efficacy (DURABLE) trial 24-week results: safety and efficacy of insulin lispro mix 75/25 versus insulin glargine added to oral antihyperglycemic drugs in patients with type 2 diabetes. *Diabetes Care.* 2009;32(6):1007-1013.

111. Holman RR, Thorne KI, Farmer AJ, et al. Addition of biphasic, prandial, or basal insulin to oral therapy in type 2 diabetes. *N Engl J Med.* 2007;357(17):1716-1730.

112. Raslova K, Bogoev M, Raz I, Leth G, Gall MA, Hancu N. Insulin detemir and insulin aspart: a promising basal-bolus regimen for type 2 diabetes. *Diabetes Res Clin Pr.* 2004;66(2):193-201.

113. Williams-Herman D, Johnson J, Teng R, et al. Efficacy and safety of initial combination therapy with sitagliptin and metformin in patients with type 2 diabetes: a 54-week study. *Curr Med Res Opin.* 2009;25(3):569-583.

114. Lee WC, Balu S, Cobden D, Joshi AV, Pashos CL. Medication adherence and the associated health-economic impact among patients with type 2 diabetes mellitus converting to insulin pen therapy: an analysis of third-party managed care claims data. *Clin Ther.* 2006;28(10):1712-1725; discussion 1710-1711.

115. Goh HK, Chew DEK, Miranda IG, Tan L, Lim GH. 24-Hour observational ward management of diabetic patients presenting with hypoglycaemia: a prospective observational study. *Emerg Med J.* 2009;26(10):719-723.

116. Gurlek A, Erbas T, Gedik O. Frequency of severe hypoglycaemia in type 1 and type 2 diabetes during conventional insulin therapy. *Exp Clin Endocr Diab.* 1999;107(3):220-224.

117. Panikar V, Chandalia HB, Joshi SR, Fafadia A, Santvana C. Beneficial effects of triple drug combination of pioglitazone with glibenclamide and metformin in type 2 diabetes mellitus patients on insulin therapy. *J Assoc Physician India.* 2003;51:1061-1064.

118. Rhoads GG, Orsini LS, Crown W, Wang S, Getahun D, Zhang Q. Contribution of hypoglycemia to medical care expenditures and short-term disability in employees with diabetes. *J Occup Environ Med.* 2005;47(5):447-452.

119. Alvarez-Guisasola F, Yin DD, Nocea G, Qiu Y, Mavros P. Association of hypoglycemic symptoms with patients' rating of their health-related quality of life state: a cross sectional study. *Health Qual Life Out.* 2010;8:86.

120. Davis RE, Morrissey M, Peters JR, Wittrup-Jensen K, Kennedy-Martin T, Currie CJ. Impact of hypoglycaemia on quality of life and productivity in type 1 and type 2 diabetes. *Curr Med Res Opin.* 2005;21(9):1477-1483.

121. Harsch IA, Stocker S, Radespiel T, et al. Traffic hypoglycaemias and accidents in patients with diabetes mellitus treated with different antidiabetic regimens. *J Intern Med.* 2002;252(4):352-360.

122. Hermanns N, Kulzer B, Krichbaum M, Kubiak T, Haak T. Affective and anxiety disorders in a German sample of diabetic patients: prevalence, comorbidity and risk factors. *Diabet Med.* 2005;22(3):293-300.

123. Labad J, Price JF, Strachan MWJ, et al. Symptoms of depression but not anxiety are associated with central obesity and cardiovascular disease in people with type 2 diabetes: the Edinburgh Type 2 Diabetes Study. *Diabetologia.* 2010;53(3):467-471.

124. Leiter L YJ-F, Chiason J-L, Harris S, Kleinstiver P, Saauriol L. Assessment of the impact of fear of hypoglycemic episodes on glycemic and hypoglycemia management. *Can J Diabetes.* 2005;29(3):1-7.

125. Lundkvist J, Berne C, Bolinder B, Jonsson L. The economic and quality of life impact of hypoglycemia. *Eur J of Health Econ.* 2005;6(3):197-202.

126. Vexiau P, Mavros P, Krishnarajah G, Lyu R, Yin D. Hypoglycaemia in patients with type 2 diabetes treated with a combination of metformin and sulphonylurea therapy in France. *Diabetes Obes Metab.* 2008;10 Suppl 1:16-24.

127. Ben-Ami H, Nagachandran P, Mendelson A, Edoute Y. Drug-induced hypoglycemic coma in 102 diabetic patients. *Arch Intern Med.* 1999;159(3):281-284.

128. Greco D, Pisciotta M, Gambina F, Maggio F. Severe hypoglycaemia leading to hospital admission in type 2 diabetic patients aged 80 years or older. *Exp Clin Endocr Diab.* 2010;118(4):215-219.

129. Redelmeier DA, Kenshole AB, Ray JG. Motor vehicle crashes in diabetic patients with tight glycemic control: a population-based case control analysis. *PLoS Med* 2009;6(12):e1000192.

130. Stork ADM, van Haeften TW, Veneman TF. The decision not to drive during hypoglycemia in patients with type 1 and type 2 diabetes according to hypoglycemia awareness. *Diabetes Care.* 2007;30(11):2822-2826.

131. Zargar AH, Wani AI, Masoodi SR, et al. Causes of mortality in diabetes mellitus: data from a tertiary teaching hospital in India. *Postgrad Med.* 2009;85(1003):227-232.

132. Dailey G, Strange P, Riddle M. Reconsideration of severe hypoglycemic events in the treat-to-target trial. *Diabetes Tech Ther.* 2009;11(8):477-479.

133. Cobden D, Lee WC, Balu S, Joshi AV, Pashos CL. Health outcomes and economic impact of therapy conversion to a biphasic insulin analog pen among privately insured patients with type 2 diabetes mellitus. *Pharmacotherapy.* 2007;27(7):948-962.

134. Daly P KL, Lorber D. *FMCSA Expert Panel Commentary and Recommendations: Diabetes and CMV Drive Safety* 2006.

135. Hemmelgarn B, Levesque LE, Suissa S. Anti-Diabetic Drug Use and the Risk of Motor Vehicle Crash in the Elderly. *Can J Clin Pharmacol.* 2006;13(1):e112-e120.

136.   Aschner P, Kipnes MS, Lunceford JK, et al. Effect of the dipeptidyl peptidase-4 inhibitor sitagliptin as monotherapy on glycemic control in patients with type 2 diabetes. *Diabetes Care.* 2006;29(12):2632-2637.

137.   Bennett WL, Maruthur NM, Singh S, et al. Comparative effectiveness and safety of medications for type 2 diabetes: an update including new drugs and 2-drug combinations. *Ann Intern Med.* 3 2011;154(9):602-613.

138.   Qayyum R, Bolen S, Maruthur N, et al. Systematic review: comparative effectiveness and safety of premixed insulin analogues in type 2 diabetes. *Ann Intern Med.* 2008;149(8):549-559.

139.   Feil DG, Rajan M, Soroka O, Tseng CL, Miller DR, Pogach LM. Risk of hypoglycemia in older veterans with dementia and cognitive impairment: implications for practice and policy. *J Am Geriatr Soc.* 2011;59(12):2263-2272.

140.   Unger J, Parkin C. Hypoglycemia in insulin-treated diabetes: a case for increased vigilance. *Postgrad Med.* 2011;123(4):81-91.

141.   Amiel SA, Dixon T, Mann R, Jameson K. Hypoglycaemia in Type 2 diabetes. *Diabet Med.* 2008;25(3):245-254.

142.   Graveling AJ, Frier BM. Hypoglycaemia: an overview. *Prim Care Diabetes.* 2009;3(3):131-139.

143.   Cryer PE. Diverse causes of hypoglycemia-associated autonomic failure in diabetes. *N Engl J Med.* 2004;350(22):2272-2279.

144.   Banarer S, Cryer PE. Hypoglycemia in type 2 diabetes. *Med Clin North Am.* 2004;88(4):1107-1116.

145.   Biesenbach G, Raml A, Schmekal B, Eichbauer-Sturm G. Decreased insulin requirement in relation to GFR in nephropathic Type 1 and insulin-treated Type 2 diabetic patients. *Diabet Med.* 2003;20(8):642-645.

146.   Snyder RW, Berns JS. Use of insulin and oral hypoglycemic medications in patients with diabetes mellitus and advanced kidney disease. *Semin Dial.* 2004;17(5):365-370.

147.   Weir MA, Gomes T, Mamdani M, et al. Impaired renal function modifies the risk of severe hypoglycaemia among users of insulin but not glyburide: a population-based nested case-control study. *Nephol Dial Transpl.* 2011;26(6):1888-1894.

148.   Punthakee Z, Miller ME, Launer LJ, et al. Poor cognitive function and risk of severe hypoglycemia in type 2 diabetes: Post hoc epidemiologic analysis of the ACCORD trial. *Diabetes Care.* 2012;35(4):787-793.

149.   Holt P. Taking hypoglycaemia seriously: diabetes, dementia and heart disease. *Br J Community Nurs.* 2011;16(5):246-249.

150.   Croxson. Hypoglycaemia, cognition and the older person with diabetes. *Prat Diab Int.* 2010;27(6):219-220.

151.   Akram K, Pedersen-Bjergaard U, Borch-Johnsen K, Thorsteinsson B. Frequency and risk factors of severe hypoglycemia in insulin-treated type 2 diabetes: a literature survey. *J Diabetes Complicat.* 2006;20(6):402-408.

152.   Bulsara MK, Holman CD, Davis EA, Jones TW. Evaluating risk factors associated with severe hypoglycaemia in epidemiology studies-what method should we use? *Diabet Med.* 2004;21(8):914-919.

153.   Wright RJ, Frier BM. Vascular disease and diabetes: is hypoglycaemia an aggravating factor? *Diabetes Metab Res Rev.* 2008;24(5):353-363.

154.   Desouza CV, Bolli GB, Fonseca V. Hypoglycemia, diabetes, and cardiovascular events. *Diabetes Care.* 2010;33(6):1389-1394.

155.   Yakubovich N, Gerstein HC. Serious cardiovascular outcomes in diabetes: the role of hypoglycemia. *Circulation.* 2011;123(3):342-348.

156.   Johnston SS, Conner C, Aagren M, Smith DM, Bouchard J, Brett J. Evidence linking hypoglycemic events to an increased risk of acute cardiovascular events in patients with type 2 diabetes. *Diabetes Care.* 2011;34(5):1164-1170.

157.   Moore TJ, Cohen MR, Furberg CD. Serious adverse drug events reported to the Food and Drug Administration, 1998-2005. *Arch Intern Med.* 2007;167(16):1752-1759.

158.   Kosiborod M, Inzucchi SE, Goyal A, ct al. Relationship between spontaneous and iatrogenic hypoglycemia and mortality in patients hospitalized with acute myocardial infarction. *JAMA.* 2009;301(15):1556-1564.

159.   Warren RE, Frier BM. Hypoglycaemia and cognitive function. *Diabetes Obes Metab.* 2005;7(5):493-503.

160.   Reijmer YD, van den Berg E, Ruis C, Kappelle LJ, Biessels GJ. Cognitive dysfunction in patients with type 2 diabetes. *Diabetes Metab Res Rev.* 2010;26(7):507-519.

161.   MacLeod KM. Diabetes and driving: towards equitable, evidence-based decision-making. *Diabet Med.* 1999;16(4):282-290.

162.   Jacobson AM, Musen G, Ryan CM, et al. Long-term effect of diabetes and its treatment on cognitive function. *N Engl J Med.* 2007;356(18):1842-1852.

163.   Launer LJ, Miller ME, Williamson JD, et al. Effects of intensive glucose lowering on brain structure and function in people with type 2 diabetes (ACCORD MIND): a randomised open-label substudy. *Lancet Neurol.* 2011;10(11):969-977.

164.   Aung PP, Strachan MW, Frier BM, Butcher I, Deary IJ, Price JF. Severe hypoglycaemia and late-life cognitive ability in older people with Type 2 diabetes: the Edinburgh Type 2 Diabetes Study. *Diabet Med.* 2012;29(3):328-336.

165. Strachan MW, Reynolds RM, Frier BM, Mitchell RJ, Price JF. The relationship between type 2 diabetes and dementia. *Br Med Bull.* 2008;88(1):131-146.

166. Fitzpatrick D, Duncan EA. Improving post-hypoglycaemic patient safety in the prehospital environment: a systematic review. *Emerg Med J.* 2009;26(7):472-478.

167. Budnitz DS, Shehad N, Kegler SR, Richards CL. Medication use leading to emergency department visits for adverse drug events in older adults. *Ann Intern Med.* 2007;147(11):755-765.

168. Budnitz DS, Lovegrove MC, Shehab N, Richards CL. Emergency hospitalizations for adverse drug events in older Americans. *N Engl J Med.* 2011;365(21):2002-2012.

169. Barendse S, Singh H, Frier BM, Speight J. The impact of hypoglycaemia on quality of life and related patient-reported outcomes in Type 2 diabetes: a narrative review. *Diabet Med.* 2012;29(3):293-302.

170. Biessels GJ. Intensive glucose lowering and cognition in type 2 diabetes. *Lancet Neurol.* 2011;10(11):949-950.

171. Barnett AH, Krentz AJ, Strojek K, et al. The efficacy of self-monitoring of blood glucose in the management of patients with type 2 diabetes treated with a gliclazide modified release-based regimen. A multicentre, randomized, parallel-group, 6-month evaluation (DINAMIC 1 study). *Diabetes Obes Metab.* 2008;10(12):1239-1247.

172. Bolli G, Dotta F, Rochotte E, Cohen SE. Efficacy and tolerability of vildagliptin vs. pioglitazone when added to metformin: a 24-week, randomized, double-blind study. *Diabetes Obes Metab.* 2008;10(1):82-90.

173. Bolli G, Dotta F, Colin L, Minic B, Goodman M. Comparison of vildagliptin and pioglitazone in patients with type 2 diabetes inadequately controlled with metformin. *Diabetes Obes Metab.* 2009;11(6):589-595.

174. Dormandy JA, Charbonnel B, Eckland DJA, et al. Secondary prevention of macrovascular events in patients with type 2 diabetes in the PROactive Study (PROspective pioglitAzone Clinical Trial In macroVascular Events): a randomised controlled trial. *Lancet.* 2005;366(9493):1279-1289.

175. Marre M, Shaw J, Br, et al. Liraglutide, a once-daily human GLP-1 analogue, added to a sulphonylurea over 26 weeks produces greater improvements in glycaemic and weight control compared with adding rosiglitazone or placebo in subjects with Type 2 diabetes (LEAD-1 SU). *Diabetic Med.* 2009;26(3):268-278.

176. Meneghini LF, Rosenberg KH, Koenen C, Merilainen MJ. Insulin detemir improves glycaemic control with less hypoglycaemia and no weight gain in patients with type 2 diabetes who were insulin naive or treated with NPH or insulin glargine: clinical practice experience from a German subgroup of the PREDICTIVE study. *Diabetes Obes Metab.* 2007;9(3):418-427.

177.   Nauck MA, Meininger G, Sheng D, Terranella L, Stein PP, Sitagliptin Study G.
Efficacy and safety of the dipeptidyl peptidase-4 inhibitor, sitagliptin, compared with
the sulfonylurea, glipizide, in patients with type 2 diabetes inadequately controlled on
metformin alone: a randomized, double-blind, non-inferiority trial. *Diabetes Obes Metab.*
2007;9(2):194-205.

178.   Olansky L, Reasner C, Seck TL, et al. A treatment strategy implementing combination
therapy with sitagliptin and metformin results in superior glycaemic control versus
metformin monotherapy due to a low rate of addition of antihyperglycaemic agents.
Diabetes Obes Metab. 2011;13(9):841-849.

179.   Pratley RE, Nauck M, Bailey T, et al. Liraglutide versus sitagliptin for patients with type
2 diabetes who did not have adequate glycaemic control with metformin: a 26-week,
randomised, parallel-group, open-label trial. *Lancet.* 2010;375(9724):1447-1456.

180.   Standl E, Maxeiner S, Raptis S, Group HOES. Once-daily insulin glargine administration
in the morning compared to bedtime in combination with morning glimepiride in
patients with type 2 diabetes: an assessment of treatment flexibility. *Hormone Metab Res.*
2006;38(3):172-177.

181.   Goldstein BJ, Feinglos MN, Lunceford JK, Johnson J, Williams-Herman DE, Sitagliptin
036 Study G. Effect of initial combination therapy with sitagliptin, a dipeptidyl
peptidase-4 inhibitor, and metformin on glycemic control in patients with type 2 diabetes.
Diabetes Care. 2007;30(8):1979-1987.

182.   Zinman B, Gerich J, Buse JB, et al. Efficacy and safety of the human glucagon-like
peptide-1 analog liraglutide in combination with metformin and thiazolidinedione in
patients with type 2 diabetes (LEAD-4 Met+TZD). *Diabetes Care.* 2009;32(7):1224-
1230.

183.   Quilliam BJ, Simeone JC, Ozbay AB, Kogut SJ. The incidence and costs of
hypoglycemia in type 2 diabetes. *Am J Manag Care.* 2011;17(10):673-680.

184.   Charbonnel B, DeFronzo R, Davidson J, et al. Pioglitazone use in combination with
insulin in the prospective pioglitazone clinical trial in macrovascular events study
(PROactive19). *J Clin Endocrinol Metab.* 2010;95(5):2163-2171.

185.   Drouin P. Diamicron MR once daily is effective and well tolerated in type 2 diabetes: a
double-blind, randomized, multinational study. *J Diabetes Complicat.* 2000;14(4):185-
191.

186.   Abraira C, Duckworth W, McCarren M, et al. Design of the cooperative study on
glycemic control and complication in diabetes mellitus type 2 Veterans Affairs Diabetes
Trial. *J Diabetes Complicat.* 2003;17:314-322.

187.   Garber A, Henry R, Ratner R, et al. Liraglutide versus glimepiride monotherapy for type
2 diabetes (LEAD-3 Mono): a randomised, 52-week, phase III, double-blind, parallel-
treatment trial. *Lancet.* 2009;373(9662):473-481.

188. Hypertension in Diabetes Study IV. Therapeutic requirements to maintain tight blood pressure control. *Diabetologia.* 1996;39(12):1554-1561.

189. Rosenstock J, Ahmann AJ, Colon G, Scism-Bacon J, Jiang H, Martin S. Advancing insulin therapy in type 2 diabetes previously treated with glargine plus oral agents: prandial premixed (insulin lispro protamine suspension/lispro) versus basal/bolus (glargine/lispro) therapy. *Diabetes Care.* 2008;31(1):20-25.

190. U.K.Hypoglycaemia Study Group. Risk of hypoglycaemia in types 1 and 2 diabetes: effects of treatment modalities and their duration. *Diabetologia.* 2007;50:1140-1147.

191. UKPDS 28: a randomized trial of efficacy of early addition of metformin in sulfonylurea-treated type 2 diabetes. U.K. Prospective Diabetes Study Group. *Diabetes Care.* 1998;21(1):87-92.

APPENDIX A. SEARCH STRATEGY

Database: Ovid MEDLINE(R)
Search Strategy:

----

1   exp Hypoglycemia/ or hypoglycemia.mp.
2   exp Diabetes Mellitus, Type 2/ or type 2 diabetes.mp.
3   1 and 2
4   limit 3 to (english language and humans)
5   limit 4 to (addresses or bibliography or biography or dictionary or directory or duplicate publication or editorial or interview or introductory journal article or lectures or legal cases or legislation or letter or news or newspaper article or patient education handout or portraits or comment or historical article or interview or case reports)
6   4 not 5
7   limit 6 to "all child (0 to 18 years)"
8   limit 6 to "all adult (19 plus years)"
9   7 not 8
10 6 not 9

NOTE: an additional search was performed using the British spelling (hypoglycaemia) as a title/abstract word

APPENDIX B. CRITERIA USED IN QUALITY ASSESSMENT OF NON-RANDOMIZED STUDIES

We evaluated each non-randomized trial based on the five elements below. To be considered low risk of bias for any element, a "yes" response was required for each of the questions (a, b, c) pertaining to the element, if applicable. Plots were developed to show the percent of the non-randomized trials in each area (human resources practices, organizational culture, and physical environment) that were assigned a yes (met criteria) or no (failed to meet criteria) for each element.

1) **Population**
   a. Is the sample representative of the population of interest?
   b. Did researchers apply inclusion/exclusion criteria uniformly to all comparison groups and is the selection of the comparison group appropriate?
   c. Is the sampling method appropriate (i.e., appropriate database or sample for research question, adequate response rate for survey studies, etc.)?

2) **Outcomes**
   a. Are important outcomes assessed and *reported* (i.e., not just intermediate or surrogate outcomes)?
   b. Was the length of follow-up appropriate for the research questions (consider benefits and harms)?
   c. Is the impact of loss to follow-up (or differential loss to follow-up) considered in the analysis?

3) **Measurement**
   a. Are outcome, predictor and covariates assessed in the same way for everyone?
   b. Is this blinded such that, for example, a person's exposure status would not be known at the time outcome status was assessed? This is where recall bias and other types of differential assessment come into play.
   c. Are the tools used to assess exposures and outcomes accurate and reliable (i.e., are standard measures used)?

4) **Confounding**
   a. Are the statistical methods and study design adequate for minimizing confounding?
   b. Aside from the exposure of interest, are groups balanced in terms of factors that might bias the exposure and outcome association?
   c. Are the appropriate confounding factors included in the analysis?

5) **Intervention (if applicable)**
   a. Is the intervention clearly described and transferrable (i.e., could someone else repeat this study with different staff and patients and get similar results)?

APPENDIX C. PEER REVIEW COMMENTS/AUTHOR RESPONSES

REVIEWER COMMENT	RESPONSE
1. Are the objectives, scope, and methods for this review clearly described?	
Yes	
Yes	
Yes For the most part the scope/methods are clearly articulated and relatively easy to follow. A couple minor points that may warrant clarification in the methods:	We moved the definition of severe hypoglycemia to the Methods section. We chose to exclude studies with fewer than 500 subjects and less than 26 weeks' duration for feasibility; as it is we abstracted 60 studies for KQ1. As suggested, we included the rationale and methods for KQ1-extension in the Methods Section. We revised the executive summary background and the analytic framework as recommended.
1) Though the results clearly delineate how each study defined severe hypoglycemia, I did not see the review methods specify how you were defining "severe hypoglycemia" for the purposes of study selection – I got the sense from results that you were very inclusive and left the definitions up to each study, but this would be worth stating explicitly in the methods. I also inferred from results that study had to essentially report incidence of symptomatic hypoglycemia – again, worth stating in methods. Also, what if the study did not explicitly define "severe hypoglycemia" but rather just presented incidences of glucose < 40 or < 60 or < 70? I assume these studies would be excluded because there was no mention of symptoms/need for assistance?	
2) What is the rationale for excluding studies of duration < 6 mos? Severe hypoglycemia is not really a time-dependent phenomenon (though the consequences of it may be). In any case, this is probably a moot point given the supplemental search, but may be worth more clearly defining rationale here. Also, the KQ1 "extension" is not mentioned in the methods, but then is presented in flow diagram – this may be confusing for readers and may want to include "extension" rationale and methods in the Methods section.	
Introduction – small point – the exec summ background paragraph states intensive control only associated with reduction in microalbuminuria while the introduction in body of paper more properly states the broader impact of intensive control (esp since these include UKPDS) on other microvascular outcomes.	
Analytic framework – the one thing that seems to be missing from this is patient behaviors – certainly things like exercise, inconsistent meals, medication mishandling etc would contribute to risk. I doubt these things are identified in any of the included studies, but the lack of such evidence may still be important to know about.	
No Although this dichotomous question requires a yes/no answer, neither is really correct. The review fails to put the issue of hypoglycemia in proper context. There is considerable variation in the definitions applied in studies of hypoglycemia. This variation and controversy surrounding it is important background. In addition, although a very explicit definition of severe hypoglycemia was chosen, there is a serious limitation as far as answering the Key Question #1: What is the incidence of clinically significant hypoglycemia? Their definition of severe hypoglycemia chosen was: "an episode with typical symptoms (e.g., sweating, dizziness, tremor, visual disturbance) that resolves after treatment (oral carbohydrate, intramuscular glucagon, or intravenous glucose) administered by another person." There is clinically significant hypoglycemia that does not meet this definition. In addition, it does not address the issue of hypoglycemia unawareness which can result in unrecognized and untreated hypoglycemia with levels of glucose <40 mg/dl. (Compare reported rates to those reported on CGMS)	We agree that there is clinically significant hypoglycemia that does not meet our definition and that asymptomatic low blood sugar (e.g., hypoglycemia unawareness) is not accounted for in this definition; however this is the definition that we chose based on its common use in the literature and that was approved by our TEP. We have acknowledged this point in our discussion.
2. Is there any indication of bias in our synthesis of the evidence?	
Yes	
Yes While there is no bias in selection of studies, from my perspective the report does not sufficiently emphasize the rates of serious hypoglycemia and possible morbidity/mortality for patients who are treated in the control arms of clinical studies or from observational data. For example, rates of potentially serious hypoglycemia in insulin treated patients was 59% in a study from a large HMO (Sarkar, 2010, Question 1). The association of serious hypoglycemia and morbidity/mortality from the standard arms of ACCORD/VADT/ADVANCE. Although observation data is not of as high quality, there are strong signals of high rates and potential harms in the selected VA populations which are not incompatible with patient self reported data. These issues are commented upon in section 4.	Although it was included in KQ3, we realized that Sarkar et al. 2010 should have been included in KQ1 ext and added it. Thank you.

REVIEWER COMMENT	RESPONSE
Yes I understand that large trials are needed to detect outcomes (i.e. severe hypoglycemia) that occur relatively infrequently. However, there were many trials with 400-499 patients with T2DM that reported the incidence of severe hypoglycemia. Some of these trials were part of the drug development program for the agent. What was the reasoning behind selecting the 500 patient cut-off? I am concerned that omitting these trials could introduce bias?	See previous page, first response.
No	
Yes Although this dichotomous question requires a yes/no answer, neither is really correct. My concern the way the results are presented and the use of the word "low" as in the following: "Overall incidence of severe hypoglycemia was low in the vast majority of the 60 reviewed studies, particularly those of metformin (0-1.5%), glucagon-like peptide-1 GLP-1 analogs (< 1%), dipeptidyl-peptidase-4 (DPP-4) inhibitors (<1%), insulin detemir (<1%), insulin aspartame (<1%), glinides (0%) and thiazolidinediones (TZDs) (<1%). Annual rates of severe hypoglycemia were greater than 1% for sulfonylureas and the following insulin preparations: neutral protamine Hagedorn (NPH), glargine, lispro and gluisine." "Low" is in the eye of the beholder. When up to 18% of patients on insulin report an episode of hypoglycemia requiring assistance in the previous year, that doesn't sound low. I do, however, appreciate consideration of additional studies "to gain a broader population-based perspective on incidence of symptomatic hypoglycemia."	We agree that use of the term "low" to describe the frequency of severe hypoglycemia is a value judgment and we have either removed or modified that term in the final report.
No	
3. Are there any published or unpublished studies that we may have overlooked?	
Yes Feil DG, Rajan M, Soroka O, Tseng CL, Miller DR, Pogach LM. Risk of hypoglycemia in older veterans with dementia and cognitive impairment: implications for practice and policy. J Am Geriatr Soc. 2011 Dec; 59(12):2263-72. Epub 2011 Dec 8. (rates of coded hypoglycemia in Veterans with cognitive impairment or dementia Seaquist ER, Miller ME, Bonds DE, Feinglos M, Goff DC Jr, Peterson K, Senior P; for the ACCORD Investigators. The Impact of Frequent and Unrecognized Hypoglycemia on Mortality in the ACCORD Study. Diabetes Care. Rhoads GG, Orsini LS, Crown W, Wang S, Getahun D, Zhang Q. Contribution of hypoglycemia to medical care expenditures and short-term disability in employees with diabetes. J Occup Environ Med. 2005 May; 47(5):447-52. Diabetes Care. 2012 Feb; 35(2):409-414. Epub 2011 Dec 16.	We thank the reviewers for bringing these articles to our attention. Of these, 3 were published after November 2011 which is when our last literature search was performed (Bonds, Feil, Seaquist); 2 had been excluded due to the fact that severe hypoglycemia was not defined (Raz, Swinnen); one we had already included (Rhoads), one was a duplicate publication of a study already included (Miser); one was a study of a newer agent approved by the FDA after our study was initiated (Owens); two meet our criteria, were not previously reviewed and have been added to our final report in KQ1 (Nauck, Russell Jones).

REVIEWER COMMENT	RESPONSE
I randomly selected a few of the drugs (lispro, detemir, linagliptin, and liraglutide) and searched PubMed to see if there were other relevant articles. I came across the following articles that were >500 patients, ≥ 6 months, and presented data on severe hypoglycemia. It is not clear to me why these studies were excluded.	See comment above.
Raz I, et al. Effects of prandial versus fasting glycemia on cardiovascular outcomes in type 2 diabetes: the HEART2D trial. Diabetes Care. 2009 Mar;32(3):381-6.	
Miser WF, et al, Randomized, open-label, parallel-group evaluations of basal-bolus therapy versus insulin lispro premixed therapy in patients with type 2 diabetes mellitus failing to achieve control with starter insulin treatment and continuing oral antihyperglycemic drugs: a noninferiority intensification substudy of the DURABLE trial. Clin Ther. 2010 May;32(5):896-908.	
Swinnen SG, et al. A 24-week, randomized, treat-to-target trial comparing initiation of insulin glargine once-daily with insulin detemir twice-daily in patients with type 2 diabetes inadequately controlled on oral glucose-lowering drugs. Diabetes Care. 2010 Jun;33(6):1176-8.	
Owens DR, et al. Efficacy and safety of linagliptin in persons with type 2 diabetes inadequately controlled by a combination of metformin and sulphonylurea: a 24-week randomized study. Diabet Med. 2011 Nov;28(11):1352-61.	
Russell-Jones D, et al. Liraglutide Effect and Action in Diabetes 5 (LEAD-5) met+SUStudy Group. Liraglutide vs insulin glargine and placebo in combination with metformin and sulfonylurea therapy in type 2 diabetes mellitus (LEAD-5 met+SU): a randomised controlled trial. Diabetologia. 2009 Oct;52(10):2046-55.	
Nauck M, et al. Efficacy and safety comparison of liraglutide, glimepiride, and placebo, all in combination with metformin in type 2 diabetes. Diabetes Care 2009; 32: 84-90.	
No It is not specified in methods whether or not long-term consequences of inpatient hypoglycemia are considered an included study or not, but there is a study looking at long-term outcomes in patients who had had inpatient hypoglycemia: Svensson AM, McGuire DK, Abrahamsson P, Dellborg M. Association between hyper- and hypoglycaemia and 2 year all-cause mortality risk in diabetic patients with acute coronary events. Eur Heart J. 2005;26:1255-61.	This article was not included because it focused on inpatients.
No	
1) More recent reports from ACCORD should be included, notably the ACCORD-EYE study and the ACCORD-MIND study, which showed reduction of retinopathy and reduction of brain shrinkage with intensive control of type 2 diabetes. 2) Include the 3 year results of the 4T study: Holman RR et al. NEJM 2009;361:1736-47 3) In addition to the report by Zoungas on associations of hypoglycemia with mortality risk, consider: Kosiborod M et al. JAMA 209;301:1556-64 and Boucai L et al. Am J Med 2011;124: 1028-35	We have reviewed all the articles mentioned, none of which met our criteria for inclusion (Kosiborod, ACCORD-EYE and ACCORD-MIND) or had already been included (4T Holman). Some of these, however, have been included in the discussion.

REVIEWER COMMENT	RESPONSE
4. Additional suggestions or comments	
From my perspective, the literature supports the following logic sequence that is relevant to VHA patient safety issues which I do not believe come thru in recommendations of the report. 1. Based upon randomized trials of medications, most of which are industry funded and of shorter duration, serious hypoglycemia is uncommon, even in insulin treated patients. 2. The recent ACCORD, VADT, ADVANCE studies were consistent in that while serious hypoglycemia was more common in the intensive arm, the health impact was greater in the standard arm for cardiovascular morbidity, and mortality (Zoungas NEJM 2010, Bonds DE BMJ 2010, Davis SJ (abstract, 2009), as well as with increased medical assistance (Miller et al BMJ 2010). The adjusted strength of association in the standard group in Accord was 2.87 (1.73 to 4.76); ADVANCE death from a cardiovascular cause (hazard ratio, 2.68; 95% CI, 1.72 to 4.19), VADT is not published, but the OR for recurrent severe hypoglycemia and mortality was 3.7. Although the recent article by Bonds et al (2012) found that prior episodes of serious hypoglycemia attenuated the association between hypoglycemia and mortality, it did not do so in the control arm. While it is not likely that this issue will even be conclusively resolved, the reviewer concludes that hypoglycemia is a strong risk factor for cardiovascular death in patients who are not "intensively treated" 3. The risk factors for serious hypoglycemia are varied and differ across the studies, but include other medical conditions, minority status, neuropathy, cognitive impairment, limited health literacy. Although causality of hypoglycemia upon adverse outcomes cannot be proven, the results from the 3 major trials would clearly indicate that Veterans at high risk for serious hypoglycemia can be identified. 4. The studies underestimate the risk of severe hypoglycemia in general practice, particularly for insulin treatment. A surveillance studies in an HMO (Sarkar 2010) noted that 59% of patients on insulin reported a significant hypoglycemia within a year. The Budnitz 2010 study, which will be included after review, will underscore that insulin and sulfonylurea remain high risk medications in the elderly. As noted, the Veteran literature is limited, but renal disease and cognitive impairment are two highly prevalent conditions associated with coded hypoglycemia; other factors, such as decreased health literacy, are also likely to be common in the Veteran population. The ESP did identify Moen et al. as an article documenting an association with biochemical hypoglycemia and death in Veterans with CKD. Additionally, other studies (see section 2) indicate high rates of coded hypoglycemia in Veterans with coded hypoglycemia on insulin, and in an insured population on insulin. The rates of up to 17% cited in the conclusion of Key Question 1 may thus underestimate the rates in high risk populations on insulin therapy in both insured and Veteran populations.	Most of these excellent points have been included in our revised discussion.
In several places, insulin aspart is written as insulin aspartame. Insulin aspartame is incorrect and should be corrected so that it reads insulin aspart. For the DPP-4 inhibitors, studies using vildagliptin were included (p. 95, 130-131); however, this product is not FDA approved. In the Insulin glargine (primary therapy) studies, 4/5 allowed the patient's prior oral diabetes medications to be continued (only Rosenstock 2001 did not allow concomitant oral agents). Therefore, these 4 trials were not truly primary therapy studies. On p.126 Table 3b, Buse 2011 is listed under A. Regular Insulin and Lispro Studies; Fast-short Acting. The lispro used in this study was the 75/25 mix, which is an intermediate and fasting acting mixture so it should be listed under C. Biphasic Insulin: Intermediate and fast-acting mixture.	As suggested, we changed "aspartame" to "aspart". Although vildagliptin is not FDA approved, it does appear in some of our tables because as it was included in some of the studies that also used FDA approved agents. The Buse study is now listed under "C" on Table 3B, as suggested.

REVIEWER COMMENT	RESPONSE
Nicely done, thorough report.	
My main suggestion has to do with the statement "Overall incidence of severe hypoglycemia was low in the vast majority of the 60 reviewed studies…." Though this is true, it is somewhat misleading because the subsequent summary statements do not delve into the issue of glucose targets enough. If the achieved HbA1c in 58/60 studies were 7.5% or 8% in the intervention group, the low incidence of hypoglycemia in the vast majority of studies doesn't really mean too much and it may suggest to readers that the bulk of evidence suggests that severe hypoglycemia is infrequent. I think the intensity of control really matters here and should be more clearly emphasized. It is hard to figure out from results and tables how the glucose target and/or glucose achieved relates to hypoglycemia incidence. Consider also saying more about the intensive vs less intensive evidence base in the summary statements/exec summary. Also, it might be useful to include the glucose targets for each of the studies in Table 3.	As suggested, we included an additional column in Table 1 (formerly Table 3) specifying the A1C targets and commented more extensively on the issue of intensive control in the executive summary, the summary statement, and the discussion.

We amended the statement regarding NPH vs glargine to indicate that the risk was not different, as recommended. |
| P18 – the NPH v glargine meta-analysis results are interesting. Many clinicians consider using glargine to help minimize hypoglycemia risk from NPH. I know this is not the focus of this paper, but the finding that the two drugs had equivalent risk of hypoglycemia has potential clinical importance and you could consider highlighting this more. Also, this is a pretty broad CI – I'm not sure I would say "risk is slightly higher" but not statistically significant – would probably just say no significant difference. | |
| This is a well done review of hypoglycemia from the Evidence Based Synthesis Program ESP of the V.A. The goal of ESP Centers is to generate evidence synthesis on clinical practice topics and develop clinical policies informed by evidence guide the implementation of effective services to improve patient outcomes and set the direction for future research.

The current report examines in great detail the data available on hypoglycemia in adults with type 2 diabetes. The study is well done and provides a complete, well documented compilation of current information on severe hypoglycemia and will be a major resource for investigators in the area. It will also be of use in clinical care of patients in the V.A. The methods used in the study are appropriate and comprehensive. The study will be a very useful compilation of data on hypoglycemia for future clinical studies and will be of use in defining future directions. It has some limitations in its use by non-investigators in that the limitations of the various studies are not as well delineated in an easily accessible manner for the non-expert.

Many of these limitations are mentioned throughout the document, but it would be more useful to the routine reader to have these limitations defined and a summary to help to better evaluate the data. As a simple example, many of the studies examining hypoglycemia in randomized control trials (RCTs) are obtained from pharmaceutical studies whose purpose is to establish non-inferiority of their agent against other agents in a very highly selected population. This is mentioned in the document, but again that could be lost for someone who does not read every word in the document. Another example is the use of superficially similar excellent studies, but directed at different populations and for different reasons to come to a single conclusion. One of the best examples of this are the ACCORD and ADVANCE trials, two of the best studies done on treatment of patients with type 2 diabetes but directed at different populations for different purposes. The ADVANCE study consisted of relatively mild diabetes with very few of the patients on insulin and low A1cs and ACCORD with a much more difficult population with almost half of the patients on insulin and much higher A1cs at the initiation of the study. The ACCORD trial had higher hypoglycemic numbers and consequences of treatment that may have been related to hypoglycemia which were quite detrimental.   (continued) | Thank you.

We have summarized the limitations of the data in the executive summary and the discussion. |

62

REVIEWER COMMENT	RESPONSE
(continued)	
Some of these issues of concern for the reader could be addressed in an additional summary of the limitations as mentioned above of individual studies. Another limitation of the current presentation is the difficulty in extracting clinical guidelines for care. While mentioned in the study, the clinical results in terms of outcomes of studies with high hypoglycemic rates may not justify the risk of very intensive control and perhaps standards of care could be qualified to include the risk of complications of treatment more clearly in the guideline.	
A few specific comments: Some agents used for treatment of patients with type 2 diabetes, rarely if ever cause hypoglycemia when used as individual agents in patients without severe complications. The report clearly defines most of these including metformin, DPP-4 inhibitors, glinides, etc. Some of the insulins have not been extensively tested in routine use for example detemir data are mostly derived from pharmaceutical studies carefully designed to limit the risk of hypoglycemia. Other agents such NPH or glargine have much real world data and appear to be much riskier. For true risk of hypoglycemia with agents that do not typically cause hypoglycemia, it could be useful to include studies that use these agents in combination with the hypoglycemic agents such as insulin. This might give a better view of the risk in the usual use of these agents.	
Minor Comments	
A few typographical errors are present in the manuscript, the most glaring of which is on page 4 under Conclusions–an incomplete sentence is somewhat confusing.	
Overall this is an extremely useful, carefully done, and valuable document for dissemination to professionals in practice and to researchers who will be planning future studies. I highly endorse this document and believe that it will be of great use in the V.A. and outside the V.A. for other practitioners and scientists.	

REVIEWER COMMENT	RESPONSE
1) Page 1 para 2: Microvascular complications other than albuminuria have indeed been shown: see the ACCORD-EYE study report in NEJM	1) We have re-worded the executive summary to reflect the benefits of tight control on a variety of microvascular complications
2) In Key Question #2 and elsewhere: glycated Hb is usually abbreviated as HbA1c, not HgbA1c.	2) All HgbA1C have been changed to HbA1C
3) Page 3 para 1: Here and elsewhere insulin aspart is incorrectly referred to as 'aspartame.' Aspartame is an artificial sweetener; aspart is an insulin analogue. If the computer search was done with 'aspartame' it is no wonder no significant hypoglycemia was found. It cannot be concluded that aspart does not cause severe hypoglycemia or that it differs from other rapid acting insulin analogues in this way. An excellent report including data on hypoglycemic risk with aspart is: Holman RR et al. NEJM 2009;361:1736–47. Furthermore, the main prandial insulin used in the ACCORD trial was aspart, and in the intensive arm of this trial the incidence of events requiring medical assistance was greater than 3% yearly.	4) The verbs accompanying the noun "data" are now in the plural form
4) Page 4, para 2: Here and elsewhere, 'data' is a plural noun.	5) As per our pre-determined methodology, gliclazide was not included since it is not an FDA approved medication
5) Page 9 bullet point 6: Why was gliclazide excluded from analyses? The ADVANCE trial is one of the best sources of information on long-term hypoglycemic risks, and it used gliclazide. This drug is widely used throughout the world.	6) Our discussion points out that definitions and ascertainment of hypoglycemic events varied between studies and ascertainment may have been incomplete
6) Page 9 bullet point 3: A crucial point is glossed over here. Studies were included if they reported severe hypoglycemia, but there are wide variations between studies in both definitions of severe events and (just as important) ascertainment of such events. This is the main limitation of this analysis.	7) We have corrected the spelling for Ramadan
7) Page 20 para 1: Ramadan is incorrectly spelled 'Ramadam.'	
8) Page 21 last section: This summary statement reports annual incidence of severe events greater than 1% for NPH, glargine, lispro, glulisine, and sulfonylureas. Notably missing are aspart (a leading cause of severe events in ACCORD), premixed insulin (a leading cause of events in 4T and possibly the main cause of severe events in clinical practice), and regular insulin (certainly a leading cause of events when used in sliding scales in hospital, but not tested in big clinical trials and therefore missing from this analysis). Somewhere the probably causes of these omissions should be discussed.	
9) Page 41 next to last para, which reads: "It is also possible that the robust recent findings that intense glycemic control results in a more than two-fold increase in risk of severe hypoglycemia without any clear outcomes benefits, may lead to an appropriate relaxation in HgbA1c goal levels by both clinicians and guideline developers." This statement should be amended in several ways. First, some guidelines are currently available which make the point that altering the A1c goals is appropriate for some patients, but not others. These actual guidelines should be cited for balance to this speculation. Also, the statement that there are no "clear outcomes" is incorrect. In ADVANCE and VADT, microalbuminuria was reduced. In ACCORD, microalbuminuria, retinopathy, and brain shrinkage were all reduced. In the long-term followup of UKPDS, all-cause mortality was reduced 27% in addition to microvascular events.	
5. Are there any clinical performance measures, programs, quality improvement measures, patient care services, or conferences that will be directly affected by this report? If so, please provide detail.	
Insulin was identified as a high risk medication within VHA in the high alert medication group, with a final report issued in 2009. More recently, there has been renewed discussion in OSC, PBM, and some VISNs about the need to identify Veterans who at higher risk for hypoglycemia in order to decrease potential over treatment and to improve care coordination (e.g. telehealth, post hospital discharge) for those with identified events.	
Pharmacy Benefits Management Services (PBM) along with the Medical Advisory Panel and VISN Pharmacist Executives are responsible for determining formulary status and guidance for use for pharmaceutical agents in the VA. The PBM would need to be made aware of any policies that would result from this report.	
This summary could well affect the nature of diabetes performance measurement.	
An important result of this report might be the design of prospective and structured collection of data to address the questions incompletely answered by this review of heterogenous data.	We have included this point in our discussion.

REVIEWER COMMENT	RESPONSE
6. Please provide any recommendations on how this report can be revised to more directly address or assist implementation needs.	
As noted in comment 4, the reviewer recommends that the report give greater prominence to concerns that serious hypoglycemia is an identified risk factor for morbidity in and morality in "non-intensively treated subjects" from ACCORD, ADVANCE and VADT with mean achieved A1cs of 7.5%–8.4%; rates based upon survey and administrative data indicate incidence of potential serious hypoglycemia up to 59%; and that risk factors for hypoglycemia are not uncommon among the Veteran population.	
See above responses to 1 and 2.	
1) This analysis and report are carefully done and generally confirm the findings of earlier efforts, including some important recently published data. However, the important limitations of the methods necessarily used should be included in the report. 2) One such limitation is that the endpoint in question (hypoglycemia) is rarely the primary endpoint of clinical studies, and in many cases it is not a secondary endpoint either, just an occasionally reported safety observation. Application of rigorous meta-analytic methods cannot overcome this limitation of the data provided. 3) Another limitation is that only some of the therapeutic agents commonly used have been included in the analysis. Hence, data are not available for drugs of interest. Regular insulin, for example, is a leading cause of hypoglycemia but its relative importance cannot be assessed using the present methods. 4) Two other agents which pose significant risk of severe hypoglycemia also cannot be addressed by the present methods for similar reasons: the sulfonylurea glyburide, and all forms of premixed insulin. Hypoglycemia. 5) Because of the limitations of the evidence available, few firm conclusions are possible. Rather, most of the observations are hypothesis-generating. Hence, a leading conclusion from this report should be that collection of better data, using the excellent VA data-handling system, would be very helpful.	We have included most of these points and limitations in our discussion.

APPENDIX D. STUDY QUALITY TABLES

Table 1. Individual Study Quality for KQ1, Randomized Studies

Study	Allocation concealment	Blinding	Intention-to treat analyses	Withdrawals adequately described	Quality
Abraira (VA-CSDM) 1995[30]	Unclear	Outcomes/ endpoints	No	Yes	Fair
ACCORD 2008, 2011[3, 7]	Adequate	Outcomes/ endpoints	Yes	Yes	Good
ADVANCE 2008[4]	Adequate	Outcomes/ endpoints	Yes	Yes	Good
Anderson 1997[47]	Unclear	No	Yes	No	Fair
Arechaveleta 2011[52]	Unclear	Yes (double)	Yes	Yes	Fair
Aschner 2006[136]	Unclear	Yes (double)	Yes	Yes	Fair
Aschner 2010[60]	Unclear	Yes (double)*	No	Yes	Fair
BARI 2D[58]	Unclear	Outcomes/ endpoints	Yes	Yes	Fair
Barnett 2008[171]	Adequate	No	Yes	Yes	Fair
Bolli 2008 and 2009[172, 173]	Unclear	Yes (double)	Yes	Yes	Fair
Buse 2009, 2011[36, 110]	Adequate	Outcomes/ endpoints	Yes	Yes	Good
Chou 2008[55]	Unclear	Yes (double)	No	Yes	Fair
Dailey 2004[46]	Unclear	No	Yes	Yes	Fair
Davies 2005[38]	Unclear	No	No	Yes	Fair
Dormandy (PROactive) 2005[174]	Adequate	Yes (double)*	Yes	Yes	Good
Drouin 2004[32]	Unclear	Yes (double)	No	Yes	Fair
Duckworth (VA-DT) 2009[5]	Adequate	Outcomes/ endpoints*	Yes	Yes	Good
Fritsche 2003[44]	Adequate	No	No (2 excluded)	Yes	Fair
Garber 2011[51]	Adequate	Yes (double)	No (1 excluded)	Yes	Good
Haak 2005[33]	Adequate	No	Yes	Yes	Fair
Heine 2005[42]	Adequate	No	No	Yes	Fair
Holman 2009, 2007[43, 111]	Adequate	Outcomes/ endpoints	No (1 excluded)	Yes	Good
Kendall 2005[56]	Unclear	Yes (double)	No (1 excluded)	Yes	Fair
Kennedy 2006[37]	Adequate	No	No	Yes	Fair
Liebl 2009 PREFER[48]	Unclear	No	No	Yes	Fair
Marre 2009[175]	Unclear	Yes (double)	No (1 excluded)	Yes	Fair
Matthews 2010[49]	Unclear	Yes (double)	No	Yes	Fair
Meneghini PREDICTIVE 2007[176]	Unclear	No	No	Yes	Fair
Nauck 2009[177]	Adequate	Yes (double)	No (2 excluded)	Yes	Good
Olansky 2011[178]	Unclear	Yes (double)	No	Yes	Fair
Pratley 2010[179]	Adequate	Outcomes/ endpoints	No (7 excluded)	Yes	Good
Raskin 2009[31]	Unclear	No	Yes	Yes	Fair
Ratner 2002[34]	Unclear	Yes (double)	No	Yes	Fair
Rayman 2007[45]	Unclear	No	No	Yes	Fair

Study	Allocation concealment	Blinding	Intention-to treat analyses	Withdrawals adequately described	Quality
Riddle 2003, Dailey 2009[41, 132]	Adequate	Outcomes/ endpoints	No	Yes	Fair
Rosenstock 2001[39]	Unclear	No	Yes	Yes	Fair
Rosenstock 2008[40]	Adequate	No, open-label	No	Yes	Fair
Rosenstock 2009[35]	Unclear	No	No	Yes	Fair
Russell-Jones 2009[54]	Adequate	Double*(insulin arm open-label)	No	Yes	Good
Saloranta 2002[59]	Unclear	Yes (double)	Unclear	No	Fair
Schernthaner 2004[57]	Unclear	Yes (double)	No	Yes	Fair
Seck, 2010, Nauck 2007[50, 177]	Unclear	Yes (double)	No	Yes	Fair
Standl 2006[180]	Unclear	No	No	Yes	Fair
UKPDS 33[21]	Adequate	Unclear	Yes	No	Good
Williams-Herman 2009, Goldstein 2007[113, 181]	Unclear	Yes (double)*	No	Partially	Fair
Zinman 2009[182]	Adequate	Yes (double)	No (3 excluded)	Yes	Good

*plus end points adjudicated by blinded committee

Table 2. Individual Study Quality for KQ1, Non-Randomized Studies

Study	Design	Population of interest	Outcomes assessed and reported	Measurement same for all subjects	Confounding controlled
Asche 2008[23]	Retrospective cohort	Yes	Yes	Yes	Yes
Berntorp 2011[15]	Prospective cohort	Yes	Yes	Yes	No
Bodmer 2008[24]	Retrospective cohort with nested case/ control	Yes	Yes	Yes	Yes
Davis 2010[16]	Prospective cohort	Partially*	No	Yes	Yes
Holstein 2001[17]	Prospective cohort	Yes	Yes	Yes	Yes
Leese 2003[25]	Retrospective cohort	Yes	Yes	Yes	No
Marre 2009 (PREDICTIVE)[18]	Prospective cohort	Partially*	Yes	Yes	No
Murata 2005[19]	Prospective cohort	Yes	Yes	Yes	No
Nichols 2010[26]	Retrospective cohort	Yes	Yes	Yes	No
Pencek 2009[20]	Prospective cohort	Yes	Yes	Yes	No
Quilliam 2011[183]	Retrospective cohort	Yes	Yes	Yes	Yes
Stahl 1999[28]	Retrospective case series	No	Yes	Yes	Yes
UK Hypoglycaemia Study Group[21]	Prospective cohort	Yes	Yes	No	No
Valensi 2009 IMPROVE[22]	Prospective cohort	Yes	Yes	Yes	Yes

*Included diabetes type 1

Table 3. Individual Study Quality for KQ2, Randomized and Non-Randomized Studies

RANDOMIZED CONTROLLED TRIALS					
Study	Allocation concealment	Blinding	Intention-to treat analyses	Withdrawals adequately described	Quality
ACCORD Miller 2010[89]	Adequate	Outcomes/ endpoints	Yes	Yes	Good
ADVANCE Zoungas 2010[90]	Adequate	Outcomes/ endpoints	Yes	Yes	Good

NON-RANDOMIZED TRIALS					
Study	Design	Population of interest	Outcomes assessed and reported	Measurement same for all subjects	Confounding controlled
Akram 2006[84]	Cross-sectional survey	No	Yes	No	Yes
Bruce 2009[92]	Prospective cohort	No	No	No	No
Davis 2010[16]	Prospective cohort	Partially*	No	Yes	Yes
Davis 2011[93]	Prospective cohort	Partially*	Yes	No	Yes
Duran-Nah 2008[104]	Case-control	No	Yes	Yes	Yes
Holstein 2009[102]	Case-control	No	Yes	Yes	Yes
Holstein 2011[103]	Case-control	No	Yes	Yes	Yes
Miller 2001[100]	Cross-sectional	Yes	Yes	Yes	Yes
Quilliam 2011[27]	Nested Case-control	Yes	No	Yes	Yes
Sarkar 2010[78]	Cross-sectional	Yes	Yes	No	Yes
Shen 2008[101]	Cross-sectional	Yes	Yes	Yes	Yes
Shorr 1997[97]	Retrospective cohort	Yes	Yes	Yes	Yes

*Included diabetes type 1

APPENDIX E. EVIDENCE TABLES

Table 1. Characteristics of Included Studies

Author Date Country Funding Source	Study Design Data Sources Length of Follow-up	Inclusion/Exclusion Criteria	Patient Characteristics	Intervention/ Control Target HbA1c	Definition of Severe Hypoglycemia	Study Quality
Abraira 1995[30] United States (VA Cooperative Study) Government	RCT 27 months	Inclusion criteria: Men ages 40-69, with non-insulin dependent diabetes who were being treated with insulin or judged clinically to require insulin because of failure of other therapy Exclusion criteria: Serious illness or predicted poor compliance, diagnosed >15 years prior	N=153 Age: 60.2 years % male: 100 Race/ethnicity: White=49.5 Black=24 Other=3 BMI: 31.0 Duration of diabetes: 7.8 years History of MI: 13.7% History of CHF: 2.0% History of CVA: 6.5% Current smoker: 15%	Intensive group: stepped regimen of insulin goal of HbA1c =5.1+/-1% Standard group: one or two injections of insulin/ day Goal was to avoid diabetic symptoms, excessive glycosuria, or overt hypoglycemia	Impaired consciousness requiring the help of another person, or coma, or seizure; confirmed low blood glucose concentration or rapid response to treatments expected to raise the level of blood glucose also required	Allocation Concealment: Yes Blinding: Yes Intention-to-Treat Analysis (ITT): No Withdrawals/dropouts adequately described: Yes
ACCORD 2008;[3] **Miller 2010**;[89] **ACCORD 2011**[17]; **Bonds 2009**[61] 2 countries, 77 centers Government/ industry	RCT Mean: 42 months	Inclusion criteria: type 2 diabetes and HbA1c ≥7.5%; either 40-79 years old with CV disease or 55-79 years old with significant atherosclerosis, albuminuria, LVH, or at least 2 additional risk factors for CV disease Exclusion criteria: Frequent or recent serious hypoglycemic events, unwillingness to do home glucose monitoring or inject insulin, BMI > 45, Cr > 1.5 mg/dL or other serious illness	N=10,251 Age: 62.2 years % male: 61.5 Race/Ethnicity (%): White=64.5 Black=19.0 Hispanic=7.2 BMI: 32.2 Duration of Diabetes: 10 years HbA1c: 8.3% (median)	Intensive group: Targeted an HbA1c below 6.0% Standard group: Targeted an HbA1c from 7.0% to 7.9%	Requiring medical assistance Requiring any assistance	Allocation Concealment: Yes Blinding: Outcomes assessment (endpoints) Intention-to-Treat Analysis (ITT): Yes Withdrawals/dropouts adequately described: Yes
ADVANCE 2008[4] **ADVANCE 2009** deGalan **ADVANCE 2010**[90] 20 Countries, 215 centers Government/ Industry	RCT Median: 60 months	Inclusion criteria: Diagnosis of type 2 diabetes at 30 years or older, an age of at least 55 years at the time of study entry, and a history of major macrovascular or microvascular disease or at least one other risk factor for vascular disease Exclusion criteria: Definite indication for, or contraindication to, any of the study treatments or a definite indication for long-term insulin therapy at the time of study entry	N=11,140 Age: 66 years % male: 57.5 Weight (lbs): 171.6 BMI: 28 Type 2 (%): 100 Duration of diabetes: 8.0 years HbA1c: 7.5% Aspirin: 44%	Intensive glucose control:defined as the use of gliclazide (modified release) plus other drugs as required to achieve a glycosylated Hgb value of 6.5% or less. Standard glucose control:(with target glycosylated Hgb level defined on the basis of local guidelines	Blood glucose < 2.8 mmol/L or the presence of typical symptoms and signs of hypoglycemia without other apparent cause. Severe: transient dysfunction of the CNS unable to treat themselves (i.e. requiring assistance from another person)	Allocation Concealment: Yes Blinding: Outcomes assessment (endpoints) Intention to Treat Analysis (ITT): Yes Withdrawals/dropouts adequately described: Yes

Predictors and Consequences of Severe Hypoglycemia in Adults with Diabetes – Systematic Review of the Evidence

Author Date Country Funding Source	Study Design Data Sources Length of Follow-up	Inclusion/Exclusion Criteria	Patient Characteristics	Intervention/ Control Target HbA1c	Definition of Severe Hypoglycemia	Study Quality
Akram 2006[84] Denmark Government	Cross-sectional survey (response rate: 62%) Questionnaire administered at the Steno Diabetes Center between February and May 2003	Inclusion criteria: Type 2 diabetes treated for at least one year with diet or oral glucose-lowering agents before commencement of insulin therapy. Exclusion criteria: Patients treated with sulfonylureas, ESRD, malignant disease, pregnancy, inability to complete questionnaire	N=401 Age: 66 years % male: 58 BMI: 29 Duration of diabetes: 15 years Insulin duration: 7 years HbA1c: 8.3% Impaired hypoglycemic awareness: 46%	N/A	Need for 3rd party assistance	Population: No Outcomes: Yes Measurement: No Confounding: Yes Intervention: N/A
Alvarez-Guisasola 2008[85] Europe Multicenter Industry	Cross-sectional Patient medical records and The Treatment Satisfaction Questionnaire for Medication June 2006 to February 2007	Inclusion criteria: Type 2 diabetes, age > 30 whose physicians added a SU or a TZD to metformin monotherapy between Jan 2001 and Jan 2006 and who had at least one HbA1c measure in the 12-month period before the visit date Exclusion criteria: Type 1 diabetes; pregnant women, including those with gestational diabetes; patients with diabetes secondary to other factors and patients who could not complete the questionnaire or were participating in another clinical study	N=1709 Age: 62.9 years % male: 54.9 BMI: 31.7 Duration of diabetes: 7.8 years HbA1c: 7.1% Microvascular complications: 2.2 Macrovascular complications: 26.4	N/A Target HbA1c ≤ 6.5%	Needing the assistance of others to manage symptoms or needing medical attention	Population: No Outcomes: No Measurement: Yes Confounding: No Intervention: N/A
Alvarez-Guisasola 2010[119] Seven European Countries Industry	Cross-sectional Patient medical records and The Treatment Satisfaction Questionnaire for Medication 5 years	Inclusion criteria: Type 2 diabetes, age > 30; physician added a SU or a TZD to metformin monotherapy Jan 2001 to Jan 2006 and who had at least one HbA1c measure in the 12-month period before the visit date Exclusion criteria: Type 1 diabetes; pregnant women, including those with gestational diabetes; patients with diabetes secondary to other factors and patients who could not complete the questionnaire or were participating in another clinical study	N=1709 Age: 63 years % male: 55 BMI: 31.7 Duration of diabetes: 7.84 Microvascular events: 2.2% Cardiovascular events: 26.4% HbA1c: 7.1%	N/A Target HbA1c ≤ 6.5%	Needing the assistance of others to manage symptoms or needing medical attention	Population: No Outcomes: No Measurement: Yes Confounding: No Intervention: N/A

70

Predictors and Consequences of Severe Hypoglycemia in Adults with Diabetes – Systematic Review of the Evidence

Evidence-based Synthesis Program

Author Date Country Funding Source	Study Design Data Sources Length of Follow-up	Inclusion/Exclusion Criteria	Patient Characteristics	Intervention/ Control Target HbA1c	Definition of Severe Hypoglycemia	Study Quality
Anderson 1997[47] 16 countries Industry	RCT - crossover 26 weeks	Inclusion criteria: Type 2 diabetes, ages 35-85, on insulin for at least 2 months Exclusion criteria: Other severe disease, use of beta blockers or glucocorticoids, use of insulin infusion device, severe hypoglycemia unawareness, insulin dose > 2.0U/kg or BMI > 35	N=722 Age: 59 years % male: 54 BMI: 28 Duration of Diabetes: 12.4 years Duration of insulin: 6.0 years HbA1c: 8.9%	Intervention: Insulin lispro Control: regular insulin	Episode requiring glucagon or IV glucose	Allocation Concealment: Unclear Blinding: No Intention-to-Treat Analysis (ITT): Yes Withdrawals/dropouts adequately described: No
Arechavaleta 2011[52] Multinational Industry	RCT 30 weeks	Inclusion criteria: Patients ≥18 years of age, with type 2 diabetes and with inadequate glycemic control (defined as HbA1c ≥ 6.5% and ≤9.0%) while on metformin as well as diet and exercise for at least 12 weeks prior to the screening visit Exclusion criteria: History of type 1 diabetes, used any OHA besides metformin within 12 weeks of the screening visit, had renal function impairment prohibiting the use of metformin or had a fasting finger stick glucose of <6.1 or >13.3 mmol/l at randomization	N=1035 Age: 54.9 years % male: 54.4 Race/Ethnicity (%): White=57.5 Asian=21.3 Multiracial=14.9 Other=5.2 Black or AA=1.2 Weight (lbs): 178.9 BMI: 30 Duration of diabetes: 6.8 HbA1c: 7.5%	Sitagliptin + metformin (n=516) Glimepiride + metformin (n=519)	Requiring non-medical assistance of others, and those requiring medical intervention or exhibiting markedly depressed level of consciousness or seizure	Allocation concealment: Unclear Blinding: Yes Intention to treat analysis (ITT): Yes Withdrawals/dropouts adequately described: Yes
Asche 2008[23] United States Industry	Retrospective cohort 30 weeks	Inclusion criteria: Patients with type 2 diabetes age ≥65 treated with metformin, SUs or TZDs (never having been on any of these meds before)	N=5438	SU: 58/2223 (2.6%) SU without insulin: 55/2117 (2.6%) SU with insulin: 3/106 (2.8%) metformin: 0 TZD: 20/889 (2.2%): TZD w/o insulin: 12/702 (1.7%) TZD w/ insulin: 8/187 (4.3%)	Drug-related AE defined as being coded in the database (i.e., a visit to a provider) for hypoglycemia in people who had NOT had a similar drug-related AE PRIOR to the initiation of the metformin, SU or TZD	Population: Yes Outcomes: Yes Measurement: Yes Confounding: Yes Intervention: N/A

71

Author Date Country Funding Source	Study Design Data Sources Length of Follow-up	Inclusion/Exclusion Criteria	Patient Characteristics	Intervention/ Control Target HbA1c	Definition of Severe Hypoglycemia	Study Quality
Aschner 2006[136] Multinational Industry	RCT 24 weeks	Inclusion criteria: 18-75 years old; compliant during run-in Exclusion criteria: Unstable cardiac disease, significant renal impairment, elevated AST, ALT, or CK	N=741 Duration of diabetes: 4.4 years HbA1c: 8%	Sitagliptin monotherapy:100 mg qd Sitagliptin monotherapy: 200 mg qd Placebo: qd	Loss of consciousness or requirement for medical assistance	Allocation concealment: unclear Blinding: Yes Intention to treat analysis (ITT): Yes Withdrawals/dropouts adequately described: Yes
Aschner 2010[60] Multinational 23 countries 113 sites Industry	RCT 24 weeks	Inclusion criteria: Type 2 diabetes, 18-78 years old had not been on any anti-hyperglycemic medications for at least 16 weeks with HbA1c between 6.5% and 9.0%	N=894 Age: 56 years % males: 46 BMI: 30.8 Duration of Diabetes: 2.4 years HbA1c: 7.2%	Sitagliptin 100mg qd (528) Metformin 1000 mg bid (522)	Required medical assistance	Allocation concealment: Unclear Blinding: Yes Intention to treat analysis (ITT): No Withdrawals/dropouts adequately described: Yes
Asplund 1991[105] Sweden NR	Case-control Swedish Adverse Drug Reactions Advisory Committee N/A	Inclusion criteria: Cases 19 patients with hypoglycemia (fatal or otherwise serious, unexpected, or remarkable) in patients treated with glipizide 1980-87 Controls patients on glipizide from local health care centers, matched on gender and birth date	N=19 cases Age: 75 years % male: 42 Duration of diabetes (before event): 3 years (median)	N/A	Fatal or otherwise serious, unexpected, or remarkable	Population: No Outcomes: No Measurement: No Confounding: No Intervention: N/A
BARI 2D 2009[58] Multinational 6 countries 49 sites Government/ Industry	RCT 5.3 years	Inclusion criteria: Type 2 diabetes and CAD, candidates for elective PCI or CABG. Exclusion criteria: Required immediate re-vascularization, had left main disease, Cr > 2, HbA1c > 13%, class 3 or 4 CHF, hepatic dysfunction, PCI or CABG within 12 months	N=2368 Age: 62.4 years % male: 70 BMI: 32 Type 2 (%): 100 Diabetes duration: 10.4 years Currently on insulin: 28% Baseline HbA1c: 7.7% Smoking in previous year: 22% ACE inhibitor: 77% Antithrombotic agent: 88% Beta blocker: 73%	Revascularization vs. medical therapy for CAD and insulin sensitive therapy vs. insulin therapy Target HbA1c < 7.0%	Requiring assistance with treatment and either a blood glucose level of <50 mg per deciliter or confusion, irrational or uncontrollable behavior, convulsions, or coma reversed by treatment that raises blood glucose levels	Allocation concealment: Unclear Blinding: Outcomes assessment (endpoints) Intention to treat analysis (ITT): Yes Withdrawals/dropouts adequately described: Yes

Predictors and Consequences of Severe Hypoglycemia in Adults with Diabetes – Systematic Review of the Evidence

Author Date Country Funding Source	Study Design Data Sources Length of Follow-up	Inclusion/Exclusion Criteria	Patient Characteristics	Intervention/ Control Target HbA1c	Definition of Severe Hypoglycemia	Study Quality
Barnett 2008[171] Multinational 7 countries Industry	RCT 27 weeks	Inclusion criteria: Patients with type 2 diabetes, age 40-80 years old, on OHAs with HbA1c between 7% and 10%	N=610 Age: 56 years % male: 50 Weight: 251.7 lbs BMI: 30.4 Duration of diabetes: 2.8 years	Self-monitored blood glucose(SMBG) No SMBG	Required 3d party assistance (grade 3) or required medical assistance (grade 4)	Allocation concealment: Adequate Blinding: No Intention to treat analysis (ITT): Yes Withdrawals/dropouts adequately described: Yes
Ben-Ami 1999[127] Israel NR	Case series – drug-induced hypoglycemic coma (admitted with or developed in hospital)	Inclusion criteria: Adult; nonalcoholic; nonepileptic; age 17 and older, type 2 or type 1 diabetes	N=102 Age (median): 72 years % male: 40 Type 2: 92% Duration of diabetes (median): 10 years	N/A	All patients had drug-induced hypoglycemic coma	Population: No Outcomes: Yes Measurement: No Confounding: N/A Intervention: N/A
Berntorp 2011[15] Sweden 200 sites Industry	Prospective observational 6 months	Inclusion criteria: Patients with at least one prescription for a SU, biguanide, TZD, acarbose, or prandial glucose regulator; with or without insulin use; ages 30-79	N=1154 Age: 65 years % male: 60 BMI: 29.4 Duration of Diabetes: 8.1 years HbA1c: 8.8%	N/A	Event w/ severe CNS symptoms consistent with hypoglycemia in which subject was unable to treat himself/ herself and either plasma glucose <3.1 mmol/L or reversal of symptoms upon glucagon/glucose administration	Population: Yes Outcomes: No Measurement: No Confounding: No Intervention: N/A
Bodmer 2008[24] United Kingdom Industry	Retrospective cohort with nested case control Large administrative database N/A	Inclusion criteria: At least one prescription for a SU, biguanide, TZD, acarbose, or prandial glucose regulator; with or without insulin use; ages 30-79 Exclusion criteria: Type 1 diabetes, pts with <3years data in the database before prescreen of first diabetes drug, pts with h/o ETOH, cancer, and gestational diabetes	N=50,048 Age: 60.7 years % male: 45 Case subjects: 2025 w/ recorded hypoglycemia; 73 "severe"	N/A	Mild/moderate: treated by the GP Severe: hospitalized or died	Population: Yes Outcomes: Yes Measurement: No Confounding: Yes Intervention: N/A

Author Date Country Funding Source	Study Design Data Sources Length of Follow-up	Inclusion/Exclusion Criteria	Patient Characteristics	Intervention/ Control Target HbA1c	Definition of Severe Hypoglycemia	Study Quality
Bolli 2008;[172] Bolli 2009[173] 9 countries 118 centers Industry	RCT 24 week reporting (2008) 52 week reporting (2009)	Inclusion criteria: Type 2 diabetes with HbA1c of 7.5% to 11.0% on a stable dose of metformin ≥1500 mg/day. Age 18-77, BMI 22-45, FPG < 15mmol Exclusion criteria: History of type 1 or secondary forms of diabetes; acute metabolic diabetic complications; myocardial infarction, unstable angina or coronary artery bypass surgery within the previous 6 months; CHF or liver disease	N=576 Age: 57 years % male: 63 Race/ Ethnicity (%): White=82 Hispanic=9 Asian=4 Black=3 Other=2 Weight (lbs): 200.2 BMI: 32 Type 2 (%): 100 Duration of diabetes: 6.4 years Baseline HbA1c: 8.4%	Vildagliptin 50 mg bid Pioglitazone 30 mg qd In patients on a stable metformin dose	Any episode requiring the assistance of another party	Allocation concealment: Unclear Blinding: Yes Intention to treat analysis (ITT): No Withdrawals/dropouts adequately described: Yes
Bruce 2009[92] Australia Multiple sources including industry	Prospective Cohort 1.6 years (median)	Inclusion criteria: 302 of the 587 survivors age ≥ 70 agreed to cognitive assessment in 2001; of the 246/302 who were NOT demented in 2001, 205 agreed to second assessment 18 months later	N=205 Age: 76 years Type 2 (%): 99 On insulin: 28% On SU: 45% Severe hypoglycemia: 7.2% HbA1c≤7: 46%	N/A	Episodes requiring second party assistance	Population: No Outcomes: No Measurement: No Confounding: No Intervention: N/A
Buse 2009;[110] Buse 2011[36] 11 countries 242 sites Industry	RCT 24 weeks	Inclusion criteria: Insulin naive, 30-80 years old, HbA1c>7% on at least 2 OHAs for 90 days Exclusion criteria: History of scheduled long term insulin use; recent use of other OHAs, BMI>45, recent history of severe hypoglycemia; significant hematology, oncology, renal, cardiac, hepatic, or GI disease; steroid use, pregnant or nursing	N=2091 Age: 57 years % male: 53 Race/Ethnicity (%) White=63 Asian=15 Hispanic=12 Black=6 Other=3 Weight (lbs): 195.8 BMI: 32 Type 2 (%):100 Duration of diabetes: 9.5 years HbA1c: 9.1%	Lispro mix (75/25) Glargine Added to patient's current OHA therapy which had to be maintained at current doses Target HbA1c<6.5%	Requiring assistance from another person for treatment with oral carbohydrate, intravenous glucose, or glucagon	Allocation concealment: Yes Blinding: NoIntention to treat analysis (ITT): Yes Withdrawals/dropouts adequately described: Yes Withdrawals (by group): Yes

Predictors and Consequences of Severe Hypoglycemia in Adults with Diabetes – Systematic Review of the Evidence

Author Date Country Funding Source	Study Design Data Sources Length of Follow-up	Inclusion/Exclusion Criteria	Patient Characteristics	Intervention/ Control Target HbA1c	Definition of Severe Hypoglycemia	Study Quality
Chou 2008[55] 19 countries 155 centers Industry	RCT 28 weeks January 1, 2001 to April 30th 2005	Inclusion criteria: Men and women, ages 18 to 75, type 2 diabetes, HbA1c of 7.5-12.0%, fasting C-peptide ≥ 0.8 ng/ml, FPG ≥126 mg/dl, treated with diet and/or exercise alone or who had not taken oral anti-diabetic medication or insulin for >15 days in preceding 4 months Exclusion criteria: History of severe hypoglycemia, severe edema or prior history of severe edema, prior history of hepatocellular reaction, clinically significant hepatic or renal disease, unstable or severe angina or CHF requiring pharmacological treatment, anemia, uncontrolled HTN (systolic >170 mmHg or diastolic >100 mmHg on therapy)	N=901 Age: 54.0 years % male: 58.8 Race/Ethnicity (%): White=77.3 Hispanic/Latino=9.4 Asian=7.8 Black=4.8 Other=0.7 Weight (lbs): 199.1 BMI: 31.6 Type 2 (%): 100 Duration of diabetes (median): 1.5 years Baseline HbA1c: 9.1%	1) Glimepiride (GLIM) monotherapy (1 mg OD titrated to max of 4 mg OD); n=225 2) Rosiglitazone (RSG) monotherapy (4 mg OD titrated to max of 8 mg OD); n=232 3) RSG/GLIM regimen A (4 mg/1 mg titrated to max of 4 mg/4 mg OD); n=225 4) RSG/GLIM regimen B (4 mg/1 mg titrated to max of 8 mg/4 mg); n=219 Target HbA1c: documented ≤6.5% and <7.0%	Not defined; reported results for patients with hypoglycemia receiving external assistance	Allocation concealment: Unclear Blinding: Yes Intention to treat analysis (ITT): No (1 dose required) Withdrawals/dropouts adequately described: Yes
Cobden 2007[133] United States Industry	Retrospective pre-post cohort 6 months before and 2+ years after conversion to pen device Medical and pharmaceutical claims – PharMetrics Database	Inclusion criteria: Age 18 or older, multiple diagnostic claims for type 2 diabetes, converted to BIAsp 70/30 pen for the first time; previously treated with insulin administered by syringe; data for 6 months before conversion and at least 2 years after	N=496 Age: 45.1 years % male: 56.4	N/A	Requiring emergency department visits or hospitalizations	Population: Yes Outcomes: Yes Measurement: Yes Confounding: Yes Intervention: Yes

75

Predictors and Consequences of Severe Hypoglycemia
in Adults with Diabetes – Systematic Review of the Evidence

Author Date Country Funding Source	Study Design Data Sources Length of Follow-up	Inclusion/Exclusion Criteria	Patient Characteristics	Intervention/ Control Target HbA1c	Definition of Severe Hypoglycemia	Study Quality
Dailey 2004[46] Multinational multicenter NR	Randomized, open labeled, parallel group study 26 weeks	Inclusion criteria: Established type 2 diabetes, age ≥ 18 years who had been on insulin therapy for ≥ 6 months before study with HbA1c 6-11%. Exclusion criteria: Clinically significant hepatic disease, renal impairment, a history of lactic acidosis, unstable or severe angina, known congestive heart failure (CHF, New York Heart Association class I, II, III, or IV), or uncontrolled hypertension	Age: 58.3 years % male: 52.9 Race/Ethnicity (%): Caucasian=85.4 Black=11.3 Asian=1.9 Multiracial=1.4 Hispanic Origin=6.8% BMI: 34.6 Type 2 (%):100 Duration of diabetes: 14.0 years HbA1c: 7.6%	Intervention: Glulisine subcutaneous injections 0-15 before breakfast and dinner (n=435) Comparator: RHI/NPH subcutaneous injections 30-45 before breakfast and dinner (n=441)	Severe hypoglycemia: symptomatic requiring assistance from another person and BG < 36 mg/dl or associated with prompt recovery following oral carbohydrate, IV glucose or glucagon	Allocation Concealment: Unclear Blinding: No (open-label) Intention to Treat Analysis (ITT): Yes Withdrawals/Dropouts adequately described: Yes
Davies 2005[38] Multinational Industry	RCT 24 weeks	Inclusion criteria: Type 2 diabetes sub-optimally controlled; age ≥ 18; on any OHA or insulin for > 6 months, requiring in the opinion of local MD basal long acting insulin, HbA1c > 7% and < 12%; BMI < 40 Exclusion criteria: Impaired renal function, acute or chronic metabolic acidosis; active liver disease or elevated ALT or AST; h/o hypoglycemic unawareness; diabetic retinopathy w/ recent surgery or planned surgery within 3 months; pregnancy	N=4961 Age: 58 % male: 49 BMI: 29 Type 2 (%): 100 Duration of diabetes: 12.3 years Duration of insulin use: 5.1 years	Algorithm 1: titration at every visit; managed by MD. Glargine 10 IU qhs (N=2529) Algorithm 2: titration every 3 days managed by patient (N=2504) in insulin naïve pts Glargine at a dose = to highest value of FBG in MMol over previous 7 days	Requiring assistance from another person and BG < 50 mg/dl	Allocation concealment: UnclearBlinding: No Intention to treat analysis (ITT): Partially Withdrawals/dropouts adequately described: Yes
Davis 2005[120] Wales and United Kingdom Industry	Cross-sectional survey N/A	Inclusion criteria: Patients with known type 1 or type 2 diabetes N=3200	Response rate: 861/3200 (27%) % male: 55 Type 2 (%): 69	N/A	Help from other person required	Population: No Outcomes: No Measurement: No Confounding: Yes Intervention: N/A

**Predictors and Consequences of Severe Hypoglycemia
in Adults with Diabetes – Systematic Review of the Evidence**

Author Date Country Funding Source	Study Design Data Sources Length of Follow-up	Inclusion/Exclusion Criteria	Patient Characteristics	Intervention/ Control Target HbA1c	Definition of Severe Hypoglycemia	Study Quality
Davis 2010[16] Australia Industry	Prospective Cohort Western Australia Ambulance Database and Western Australia Data Linkage System 5 years after last patient enrollment	Inclusion criteria: All patients with type 2 diabetes	N=616 Age: 67 years % male: 52.3 BMI: 28 Type 2 (%): 100 Duration of Diabetes: 7.7 years (median) HbA1c (%): Median=7.2%	Target HbA1c: N/A	Requiring ambulance attendance, emergency department services, and/or hospitalization	Population: No Outcomes: No Measurement: Yes Confounding: No Intervention: N/A
Davis 2011[93] Australia Industry	Prospective Cohort Fremantle Hospital primary catchment area with morbidity/ mortality data obtained through WA Data Linkage System 8 years	Inclusion criteria: All patients with type 2 diabetes in the Fremantle Hospital primary catchment	N=602 Age: 67.1 years % male: 52 Duration of diabetes: 7.7 years (median) HbA1c: 7.2%	N/A	Patient with a subnormal blood/ plasma/serum glucose required documented health service use (ambulance, emergency department, or hospitalization)	Population: No Outcomes: Yes Measurement: No Confounding: Yes Intervention: N/A

77

Predictors and Consequences of Severe Hypoglycemia
in Adults with Diabetes – Systematic Review of the Evidence

Evidence-based Synthesis Program

Author Date Country Funding Source	Study Design Data Sources Length of Follow-up	Inclusion/Exclusion Criteria	Patient Characteristics	Intervention/ Control Target HbA1c	Definition of Severe Hypoglycemia	Study Quality
Dormandy 2005[174] Charbonnel 2010[184] PROactive 19 countries Industry	RCT Mean: 34.5 months	Inclusion criteria: Adults (aged 35–75 yr, inclusive); type 2 diabetes; history of macrovascular disease; current use of pioglitazone or other thiazolidinediones and insulin Exclusion criteria: Monotherapy for 2 wk or longer at any time in the previous 3 months	N=5238 Age: 61.7 years % male: 66.1 Race/Ethnicity (%): White=98.6 BMI: 30.9 Type 2 (%): 100 Duration of diabetes: 9.5 years Baseline HbA1c: 8.1% Smoking: Current: 13.8% Past: 45%	Pioglitazone titrated from 15-45 Placebo Charbonel SGA an analysis of those in each randomized group who were receiving insulin at baseline *with insulin at baseline Pioglitazone (n=864) 45 U/day Placebo (n=896) *w/o insulin at baseline Pioglitazone 45 U/day Placebo	Resulting in hospital admission	Allocation concealment: Yes Blinding: Yes Intention to treat analysis (ITT): Yes Withdrawals/dropouts adequately described: Yes
Drouin 2000[185] and 2004[32] Multinational NR	RCT 10 months then 2 months during which all diamicron pts switched to diamicron MR, then 12 month open-label on diamicron MR	Inclusion criteria: Type 2 diabetes for at least 6 months, > 35 years old, BMI 22-35 treated for at least 3 months with diet with or without an OHA agent; HbA1c of 7.8% to 13.9% after washout from any previous OHA	N=507 Age: 61.5 years % male: 54 BMI: 28.5 Duration of diabetes: 6.5 years HbA1c: 8.14%	Diamicron (gliclazide) n=399 Diamicron MR (gliclazide modified release) n=401	Grade 3: required external assistance Grade 4: required medical assistance	Allocation concealment: Unclear Blinding: Yes Intention to treat analysis (ITT): No Withdrawals/dropouts adequately described: Yes

78

**Predictors and Consequences of Severe Hypoglycemia
in Adults with Diabetes – Systematic Review of the Evidence**

Author Date Country Funding Source	Study Design Data Sources Length of Follow-up	Inclusion/Exclusion Criteria	Patient Characteristics	Intervention/ Control Target HbA1c	Definition of Severe Hypoglycemia	Study Quality
Duckworth 2009[5] VA-DT[5] Abraira 2003[186] United States 20 sites Government/ Industry	RCT Median: 5.6 years	Inclusion criteria: Male and female veterans; ≥ 41 years old; nonresponsive to a maximum dose of at least one oral agent and/or daily insulin injections (centrally measured HbA1c level > 4 SD above normal mean (i.e., ≥ 7.5%) or else local HbA1c ≥ 8.3%)	N=1791 Age: 60.4 years % male: 97 Race/Ethnicity (%): White=62 Hispanic white=16.2 Black=16.7 Other=5 Weight (lbs): 214 BMI: 31.3 Type 2 (%): 100 Duration of diabetes: 11.5 years HbA1c: 9.4% Insulin: 52% Current smoker. 16%	Intensive Goal of absolute reduction of 1.5% in the HbA1c compared to standard Rx (N=892) Standard regimen One-half the max dose of intensive regimen (N=899)	Life threatening, death, hospitalization, disability or incapacity or other event requiring medical intervention/treatment	Allocation Concealment: Yes Blinding: No Intention-to-Treat Analysis (ITT): Yes Withdrawals/dropouts adequately described: Yes
Duran-Nah 2008[104] Mexico NR	Case control N/A	Inclusion criteria: Cases: consecutive patients with type 2 diabetes ≥ 30 years old, presenting to ER and hospitalized for symptomatic hypoglycemia, had to be on a diabetes medication. Controls: type 2 diabetes patients admitted for other problems	N=282 % male: 38 Age: 59 years Duration of diabetes: 13.7 years	N/A	≤ 72 mg/dL glucose concentration, with a neurological clinical picture consistent with a severely confused mental state or worse, non-arousable	Population: No Outcomes: Yes Measurement: Yes Confounding: Yes Intervention: N/A
Fadini 2009[95] Italy NR	Retrospective Cohort Chart analysis of ER visits for hypoglycemia over 6 years	Inclusion criteria: Patients type 2 diabetes presenting to ER with one of the relevant ICD9 codes Exclusion criteria: Patients with type 1 diabetes, secondary diabetes, other potential cause of coma	N=192 (126 cases included) Age: 77 years % male: 44	N/A	Led to hospitalization	Population: No Outcomes: Yes Measurement: Yes Confounding: No Intervention: N/A

Author Date Country Funding Source	Study Design Data Sources Length of Follow-up	Inclusion/Exclusion Criteria	Patient Characteristics	Intervention/ Control Target HbA1c	Definition of Severe Hypoglycemia	Study Quality
Fritsche 2003[44] 13 European countries 111 sites Industry	RCT 24 weeks	Inclusion criteria: Type 2 diabetes, <75 years old, BMI <35, previous oral therapy with any sulfonylurea or combination, FBG≥120 mg/dl, HbA1c 7.5-10.5% Exclusion criteria: Pregnancy, breast feeding, insulin or other investigational drugs in previous 3 months, clinically relevant somatic or mental diseases	N=468 Age: 61 years % male: 53.7 Duration of diabetes: 8.8 years Weight (lbs): 178.9 BMI: 28.7 HbA1c: 9.1%	Bedtime NPH, Bedtime glargine, Morning glargine All groups on 3 mg glimepiride throughout study Baseline insulin doses based on FBG; titrated at every visit Target HbA1c ≤7.5%	Symptoms consistent with hypoglycemia that require assistance of another person, associated with blood glucose <50 mg/ dL, and followed by prompt recovery with carbohydrate, IV glucose, or glucagon	Allocation concealment: Yes Blinding: No Intention to treat analysis (ITT): No Withdrawals/dropouts adequately described: Yes
Garber 2009,[187] 2011[51] United States 126 sites Mexico 12 sites Industry	RCT 52 weeks+ 52 week open label	Inclusion criteria: Type 2 diabetes, age 18-80, BMI<45, had received diet or OHA therapy (up to half of the highest dose) for at least 2 months, HbA1c between 7% and 11% (diet) or between 7% and 10% if on OHA Exclusion criteria: Insulin treatment during previous 3 months, treatment with systemic corticosteriods, hypoglycemia unawareness or recurrent severe hypoglycemia, and impaired liver function	N=746 Age: 53 years % male: 49.7 Race/Ethnicity (%): White=78.2 Black=12.6 Asian=3.5 Other=5.1 Weight: 204.4 BMI: 33.1 Duration of diabetes: 5.4 years HbA1c: 8.3%	Liraglutide 1.2 mg SC qd (251; 149 ext) Liraglutide 1.8 mg SC qd (246;154 ext) Glimepiride 8mg qd (248; 137 ext)	Major: Plasma glucose < 3.1 and required 3rd party assistance	Allocation concealment: Yes Blinding: Yes Intention to treat analysis (ITT): Yes Withdrawals/dropouts adequately described: Yes
Goh 2009[115] Singapore NR	Prospective Cohort Patient Questionnaire at the Tan Tock Seng Hospi- tal (medical records were used to fill out incomplete questionnaires) 28 days	Inclusion criteria: Patients with isolated hypoglycemia, no co-existing acute medical issue requiring a hospital stay of > 24 hours. Neurological signs and symptoms with which patients first presented must have been completely resolved with the reversal of hypoglycemia	N=203 % male: 36.9 Race/Ethnicity (%): Chinese=67.5 Malay=18.2 Indian=12.3 Other=2.0 %Type 2 diabetes: 94.6 Previous symptomatic hypoglycemia: 21.2%	N/A	Admission to the ER	Population: No Outcomes: No Measurement: No Confounding: No Intervention: N/A

Author Date Country Funding Source	Study Design Data Sources Length of Follow-up	Inclusion/Exclusion Criteria	Patient Characteristics	Intervention/ Control Target HbA1c	Definition of Severe Hypoglycemia	Study Quality
Goldstein 2007[181] Multinational Industry	RCT 24 weeks	Inclusion criteria: Ages 18 to 78, type 2 diabetes, on or not on an oral anti-hyperglycemic agent at screening Exclusion criteria: Type 1 diabetes, unstable cardiac disease, significant renal impairment, elevated liver enzymes	N=1091 Age: 53.5 years % male: 49.4 Race/Ethnicity (%): White: 51.7 Black: 6.9 Hispanic: 27.2 Asian: 5.7 Other: 8.5 BMI: 32.1 Type 2 (%): 100 Duration of diabetes: 4.5 years HbA1c: 8.8%	1) Sitagliptin 100 mg OD 2) Metformin 500 mg BID 3) Metformin 1,000 mg BID 4) Sitagliptin 50 mg + Metformin 500 mg BID 5) Sitagliptin 50 mg + Metformin 1,000 mg BID 6) Placebo All patients received counseling on diet and exercise throughout the study	Loss of consciousness or requirement for medical assistance	Allocation concealment: Unclear Blinding: Yes Intention to treat analysis (ITT): No Withdrawals/dropouts adequately described: Partially
Greco 2010[128] Italy NR	Case Series Chart analysis 8 years	Inclusion criteria: Patients admitted to the hospital with severe hypoglycemia between January 1, 2001 and December 31, 2008	N=99/5377 medical admissions due to diabetes attributed to severe hypoglycemia Age (median): 84.7 % male: 36.4 BMI: 27.8 Duration of diabetes:15.7 years	N/A	Symptomatic episode requiring assistance of another person and treatment with intravenous glucose or glucagon injection. Confirmed by blood glucose of 50mg/dl	Population: Yes Outcomes: Yes Measurement: No Confounding: No Intervention: N/A
Gürlek 1999[16] Turkey NR	Retrospective Cohort Chart Review Mean: 3.3 year	Inclusion criteria: Attended outpatient clinic weekly or biweekly for 1 year; taking conventional insulin therapy (1-2 injections), no oral medications	N=165 (baseline data reported for 114 with type 2 diabetes) Age: 58.9 years % male: 44.7 BMI: 29.8 Duration of diabetes: 12.9 years	N/A	Patient unable to take yes action themselves OR Coma requiring parenteral glucose administered in hospital setting	Population: No Outcomes: No Measurement: Yes Confounding: No Intervention: N/A
Haak 2005[33] Multinational 5 European countries 63 sites Industry	RCT 26 weeks	Inclusion criteria: Type 2 diabetes for ≥12 months, age ≥35, HbA1c in past 12 months, on insulin for ≥ 2 months Exclusion criteria: Received OHAs within 2 months of the trial; pregnant or breast feeding; proliferative retinopathy; uncontrolled hypertension; recurrent major hypoglycemia; impaired renal or hepatic function; cardiac problems; total daily basal insulin dose >100 IU/day	N=505 Age: 60.4 years % male: 51.1 Race/Ethnicity (%): White=99 Asian-Pacific Islander=1 Weight (lbs): 191.1 BMI: 30.4 Duration of diabetes: 13.2 years HbA1c: 7.9%	Detemir (341) NPH (164)	Patient unable to treat him/herself	Allocation concealment: No Blinding: No Intention to treat analysis (ITT): Yes Withdrawals/dropouts adequately described: Yes

Predictors and Consequences of Severe Hypoglycemia in Adults with Diabetes – Systematic Review of the Evidence

Author Date Country Funding Source	Study Design Data Sources Length of Follow-up	Inclusion/Exclusion Criteria	Patient Characteristics	Intervention/ Control Target HbA1c	Definition of Severe Hypoglycemia	Study Quality
Harsch 2002[121] Germany NR	Cross-sectional Anonymous questionnaire randomly distributed N/A	Inclusion criteria: Patients with diabetes (Type 1, Type 2, or unclassified); driving at least 1000 km annually, driver's license for at least 1 year, treated with potentially hypoglycemia-inducing medication for at least 1 year	**Oral Antidiabetic (OA) group** (116/122 type 2) Age: 64.2 years Duration of diabetes: 8.6 years Recent HbA1c: 7.9% Impaired visual function related to diabetes: 8.2% Antihypertensive treatment: 52.5% CNS-relevant medication: 5.7% **Conventional Insulin Therapy (CT) group** (108/151 type 2): Age: 58.8 years Duration of diabetes: 11.7 years Recent HbA1c: 7.9% Impaired visual function related to diabetes: 20.5% Antihypertensive treatment: 38.4% CNS-relevant medication: 5.3%	N/A	Patients instructed to report hypoglycemia during driving and hypoglycemia-induced accidents with hypoglycemia as a range of events from impaired psycho-physiological performance, requiring immediate self-treatment to interruption of driving events requiring external assistance	Population: No Outcomes: Yes Measurement: No Confounding: No Intervention: N/A
Heine 2005[42] 13 countries 82 centers Industry	RCT 26 weeks	Inclusion criteria: Inadequate glycemic control on max dose SU and metformin, age 30-75, HbA1c 7-10%, BMI 25-45, stable body weight Exclusion criteria: Participated in a study 30 days prior, experienced > 3 severe hypoglycemic episodes in the past 6 months, undergoing therapy for malignant disease other than basal or squamous cell skin cancer, class III or IV cardiac disease, serum creatinine > 1.5 mg/dL (men) or 1.2 mg/dL (women), symptoms of liver disease, on long term glucocorticoid therapy, prior use of weight loss drugs, treated for > 2 consecutive weeks with insulin within 3 months prior to screening	N=549 Age: 59 years % male: 56 Race/Ethnicity (%): White=80 Black=1 Asian=1 Hispanic=16 Other=2 BMI: 31 Duration of diabetes: 10 years HbA1c: 8.3%	Intervention: exenatide 5 ug bid for 4 wks then 10Ug bid till end of study Control: glargine 10U/ hs then adjusted by algorithm to achieve FBS < 100 Metformin and SU maintained at pre-study doses	Patient required assistance of another person and had a BS< 50mg/dl	Allocation Concealment: Yes Blinding: No Intention to Treat Analysis (ITT): No Withdrawals/dropouts adequately described: Unclear

82

Author Date Country Funding Source	Study Design Data Sources Length of Follow-up	Inclusion/Exclusion Criteria	Patient Characteristics	Intervention/ Control Target HbA1c	Definition of Severe Hypoglycemia	Study Quality
Hemmelgarn 2006[135] Canada NR	Nested case control N/A	Inclusion criteria: Aged 67-84 with valid driver's license in Quebec; resident for at least 2 years before June 1 1990; followed until death, end of study (May 31 1993), date of event, age 85 years, or emigration from province Exclusion criteria: Residence in a long-term care setting during the study period; previous hosp within past 60 days; hosp of 30 or more days any time in previous year	Cases: Had an injurious MVA (N=5579) Age: 74 years % male: 80 Controls: Random sample of 6% of the subjects from the cohort (N=13,300) Age 73 years % male: 73	N/A	N/A	Population: Yes Outcomes: No Measurement: No Confounding: No Intervention: N/A
Henderson 2003[76] Scotland Government/ Foundation	Cross-sectional Survey of randomly selected patients attending outpatient diabetes clinic	Inclusion criteria: Type 2 diabetes; 2 or more injections of insulin daily for at least 1 year	N=215 Age: 68 years (median)	N/A	Required external assistance to effect recovery	Population: Yes Outcomes: No Measurement: No Confounding: No Intervention: N/A
Hepburn 1993[99] Scotland NR	Cross-sectional Questionnaire given to sequentially selected patients at daily diabetic clinics (one location)	Inclusion criteria: type 2 diabetes, treated with dietary modification and oral agents for at least 2 years before start of insulin therapy; treated with insulin for at least 1 year	N=104 Age: 63 years % male: 50 BMI: 27 Duration of diabetes: 12 years Duration of insulin therapy: 4 years HbA1c: 10.5%	N/A	Patient unable to take appropriate restorative action and required assistance of another person for treatment (home or hospital) to administer either oral or parenteral glucose or glucagon by injection	Population: Yes Outcomes: Yes Measurement: No Confounding: Yes Intervention: N/A
Hermanns 2005[22] Germany NR	Cross-sectional Questionnaires given to Diabetes Center inpatients (addressed hypoglycemia in past 12 months)	Inclusion criteria: Referred for inpatient treatment (mostly for treatment of late complications or difficulty achieving glycemic control); age 18-75 yrs	N=388 (51 had severe hypoglycemia) Age: 35% 18-48 yrs, 35% 49-62 yrs, 30% >62 yrs % male: 62 Type 2: 63% Duration of diabetes: 31% <6 yrs, 37% 7-16 yrs; 32% >16 yrs HbA1c: 31% <7.5%, 34% 7.5-8.3%, 36% >8.3	N/A	Requiring assistance	Population: Yes Outcomes: Yes Measurement: No Confounding: Yes Intervention: N/A

Predictors and Consequences of Severe Hypoglycemia in Adults with Diabetes – Systematic Review of the Evidence

Author Date Country Funding Source	Study Design Data Sources Length of Follow-up	Inclusion/Exclusion Criteria	Patient Characteristics	Intervention/ Control Target HbA1c	Definition of Severe Hypoglycemia	Study Quality
Holman 2009;[43] Holman 2007[111] United Kingdom 58 sites Industry	RCT 3 years	Inclusion criteria: 18 years and older, 12 mo or longer history of diabetes, not on insulin; HbA1c 7-10% on maximal doses of metformin and SU for at least 4 months; BMI≤40; Exclusion criteria: History of TZD therapy or triple OHA therapy	N=708 Age: 61.7 years Duration of diabetes (median): 9 years	Biphasic insulin aspart bid before meals; (n=235) Prandial insulin aspart tid before meals; (n=239) Basal insulin detemir qhs (n=234)	Third party assistance required	Allocation concealment: Yes Blinding: Outcomes assessment (endpoints) Intention to treat analysis (ITT): Yes Withdrawals/dropouts adequately described: Yes
Holstein 2001[17] (subset of Holstein 2003) Germany Industry	Prospective Cohort Region of Germany with 200,000 residents 4 years	Inclusion criteria: All emergency room patients from only hospital in area (n=30,768); this publication focuses only on SU-associated hypoglycemia	N=45 Age: 83.5 years % male: 36.3 Duration of diabetes: 7.2 years BMI: 23.6 HbA1c: 5.2% Note: non-diabetic range 3.4-4.9%	N/A	Symptomatic event requiring treatment with IV glucose or glucagon and confirmed by blood glucose measurement of <2.8 mmol/L	Population: Yes Outcomes: Yes Measurement: Yes Confounding: Yes Intervention: Yes
Holstein 2003[107] Germany, Austria, Switzerland NR	Case series Cases reported by randomly chosen MDs and members of German Diabetes Assoc. at acute care hospitals	Responses received from 24/400 MDs (6%)	N=93 episodes Age: 77.7 years % male: 41 BMI: 24.7 Duration of diabetes: 9.1 years HbA1c: 5.3% Note: non-diabetic range 3.4-4.9%	N/A	Symptomatic event requiring administration of IV glucose or glucagon and confirmed by blood glucose < 2.8 mmol/l	Population: No Outcomes: Yes Measurement: No Confounding: No Intervention: N/A

Predictors and Consequences of Severe Hypoglycemia in Adults with Diabetes – Systematic Review of the Evidence

Author Date Country Funding Source	Study Design Data Sources Length of Follow-up	Inclusion/Exclusion Criteria	Patient Characteristics	Intervention/ Control Target HbA1c	Definition of Severe Hypoglycemia	Study Quality
Holstein 2003[109] Germany NR	Population-based case series N/A	Inclusion criteria: All episodes of severe hypoglycemia in all patients presenting in the emergency department of one hospital, 1997-2000	N=148 (56%) cases of severe hypoglycemia in 121 patients with type 2 diabetes Age: 76 years % male: 36 BMI: 25.7 Duration of diabetes: 17 years Renal failure (CrCl<60 ml/min): 54% HbA1c: 6.2% Note: non-diabetic range 3.4-4.9%	N/A	Symptomatic event requiring administration of IV glucose or glucagon injection that relieved symptoms and confirmed by blood glucose measurement	Population: Yes Outcomes: Yes Measurement: Yes Confounding: No Intervention: N/A
Holstein 2009[102] Germany NR	Case-control Tertiary care hospital N/A	Inclusion criteria: Type 2 diabetes, on sulfonylureas Exclusion criteria: On insulin	Cases: 43 (mean glucose level at time of event: 32) Controls: 54	N/A	Symptomatic event requiring therapy with IV glucose confirmed by blood glucose < 50 mg/dl	Population: No Outcomes: Yes Measurement: Yes Confounding: Yes Intervention: N/A
Holstein 2011[103] Germany Industry	Case-control Clinic Lippe-Detmold, a large tertiary-care hospital in East Westphalia, Germany, January 2000 -December 2009	Inclusion criteria: Patients attending the ED of Lippe-Detmold Clinic and taking sulfonylurea	N=203 Age: 78.4 years % male: 52.7 BMI: 26.9 Duration of diabetes:11.3 years HbA1c: 6.9%	Patients on sulfonylurea: Patients experiencing severe hypoglycemia (n=102) Patients with no severe hypoglycemia (n=101)	Symptomatic event requiring treatment with intravenously administered glucose and confirmed by blood glucose measurement of <50 mg/dl	Population: No Outcomes: Yes Measurement: Yes Confounding: Yes Intervention: N/A

Author Date Country Funding Source	Study Design Data Sources Length of Follow-up	Inclusion/Exclusion Criteria	Patient Characteristics	Intervention/ Control Target HbA1c	Definition of Severe Hypoglycemia	Study Quality
Honkasalo 2010[77] Finland Foundation	Retrospective Cohort Local ambulance registries, local healthcare unit databases, patient questionnaires 12 months	N/A	N=1065 patients with type 2 diabetes Age: 65.4 years	N/A	Required the help of another person to recover from a hypoglycemic episode.	Population: No Outcomes: No Measurement: No Confounding: No Intervention: N/A
Hypertension in Diabetes IV 1996[88] United Kingdom Government/ Industry/ Foundation	RCT 5 years	Inclusion criteria: Non-insulin dependent diabetes Exclusion criteria: Required strict blood pressure control or beta blockade; severe vascular disease, severe concurrent illness; pregnant women	N=758 Age: 57 years % male: 53 Race/ethnicity (%): Caucasian=87% Asian=5% Afro-Carribean=8% BMI: 29 Duration of diabetes: 3.2 years HbA1c: 6.8% Smoking: 22% current	Tight blood pressure control (<150/85 mmHg) (N=497) Less tight control (<180/105 mmHg) (N=261) Part of UKPDS	Requiring medical assistance or admission to hospital	Allocation concealment: Unclear Blinding: Unclear Intention to treat analysis (ITT): Not for hypoglycemic reactions Withdrawals/dropouts adequately described: No
Kendall 2005[56] United States 91 sites Industry	RCT 30 weeks	Inclusion criteria: Age 22-77: taking metformin and SU; FPG <13.3, BMI 27-45, HbA1c 7.5 to 11%; metformin at least 1500 mg/d and SU at maximally effect dose for 3 months; weight stable for 3 months; no abnormal labs; women postmenopausal, surgically sterile or on OCs for 3 months Exclusion criteria: Other significant medical conditions or use of other oral glucose lowering drugs or weight loss drugs within 3 months; on steroids, drugs affect GI motility, transplantation or invest drugs	N=733 Age: 56 years % male: 58 Race/Ethnicity (%): White=68 Black=11 Weight (lbs):215.6 BMI: 34 Type 2 (%):100 Diabetes duration: 8.9 years HbA1c: 8.5% ACE inhibitor: 50%	Exenatid 5ug bid N=245 Exenatide 10ug bid N=241 Placebo N=247	Required the assistance of a third party	Allocation concealment: Unclear Blinding: Yes Intention to treat analysis (ITT): Yes Withdrawals/dropouts adequately described: Yes

Predictors and Consequences of Severe Hypoglycemia in Adults with Diabetes – Systematic Review of the Evidence

Author Date Country Funding Source	Study Design Data Sources Length of Follow-up	Inclusion/Exclusion Criteria	Patient Characteristics	Intervention/ Control — Target HbA1c	Definition of Severe Hypoglycemia	Study Quality
Kennedy 2006[37] GOAL HbA1c United States 2,164 sites Industry	RCT 24 weeks	Inclusion criteria: Men and women, ≥18 years of age, diagnosis of type 2 diabetes for ≥1 year, inadequate glycemic control (A1c >7.0%) despite diet, exercise, OHAs; candidate for insulin; stable doses of current medications for ≥2 months before randomization Exclusion criteria: Severe heart failure; significant renal or hepatic disease; pregnancy or lactation; malignancy in last 5 years (except treated basal cell carcinoma); dementia; hypersensitivity to insulin glargine; any other condition that could interfere with study completion; treated with metformin with impaired renal function (modified after 498 randomized to allow continuation in study if metformin was discontinued)	N=5,721 Age: 57 years % male: 49 Race/Ethnicity (%): White=71 Black=16 Hispanic=10 Other=3 BMI: 34.3 Type 2 (%): 100 Duration of diabetes: 8.5 years HbA1c: 8.9%	1) Insulin glargine usual titration and laboratory HbA1c testing; n=1,978 2) Insulin glargine usual titration and point-of-care (POC) HbA1c testing; n=1,975 3) Insulin glargine active titration and laboratory HbA1c testing; n=1,967 4) Insulin glargine active titration and POC HbA1c testing; n=1,973	Patient required assistance and 1) there was prompt response to treatment (e.g., glucose or glucagon) or 2) SMBG level <36 mg/dl	Allocation concealment: Yes Blinding: No Intention to treat analysis (ITT): No Withdrawals/dropouts adequately described: Yes
Labad 2010[123] Scotland Government	Cross-sectional Lothian Diabetes Register 12 months	Inclusion criteria: Individuals between 60 and 74 years old with a confirmed diagnosis of type 2 diabetes Exclusion criteria: Non-type 2 diabetes, non-English speakers, or unable to read large print.	N=1066 Age: 67.9 years % male: 51.3 Race/Ethnicity (%): White=95.3 Other=4.7 Duration of diabetes: 9.1 years HbA1c: 7.4% History of severe hypoglycemia: 10.8% MI: 14.1% Angina: 28% Cerebrovascular disease: 8.7%	N/A	Needing assistance by another person	Population: Yes Outcomes: No Measurement: Yes Confounding: Yes Intervention: N/A

Author Date Country Funding Source	Study Design Data Sources Length of Follow-up	Inclusion/Exclusion Criteria	Patient Characteristics	Intervention/ Control Target HbA1c	Definition of Severe Hypoglycemia	Study Quality
Lee 2006[114] United States Industry	Retrospective pre-post cohort Medical and pharmacy claims data from PharMetrics database January 1, 2001 - April 30, 2005	Inclusion criteria: Age >18 years; multiple claims indicating a diagnosis of type 2 diabetes and use of insulin therapy; initiated treatment with insulin analogue pen device July 1, 2001 to December 31, 2002; data for at least 6 months before index date and at least 2 years of continuous enrollment after	N=1156 Age: 45.4 years % male: 53.8 Metabolic disease: 8.2% Neuropathy: 8.2% nephropathy: 7.6% retinopathy: 7.2% CVD: 6.7%	Conversion to insulin pen therapy Target HbA1c: N/A	No clear definition ED visits, hospitalizations, MD visits related to hypoglycemia	Population: Yes Outcomes: No Measurement: Yes Confounding: Yes Intervention: Yes
Leese 2003[25] Scotland Industry	Retrospective cohort DARTS/ MEMO registry N/A	Inclusion criteria: Type 1 or 2 diabetes in the registry who were alive in 1997 and who were either still alive in 1998 or had died but had not emigrated from the area during the one year study period	N=977 w/ type 1 and 7678 w/ type 2 Type 2: Age: 65 years % male: 52 Duration of diabetes: 8 years	N/A	Required emergency treatment from primary care, ambulance, or other emergency services; severe defined as blood sugar < 3.5 mmol/L requiring treatment with glucagon, IV dextrose or paramedic confirmation of low blood sugar with rapid recovery following treatment	Population: Yes Outcomes: Yes Measurement: Yes Confounding: No Intervention: N/A
Leiter 2005[124] Canada 4 sites Industry	Cross-sectional Questionnaire to patients with scheduled clinic visit	Inclusion criteria: Male or female; ages 18 years and older; type 1 or 2 diabetes; treated with insulin alone or with OHAs for at least 1 yr	N=335 (97% of patients screened) N=133 with type 2 Age: 60 years BMI: 32 HbA1c: 7.5%	N/A	Required external assistance and plasma glucose <2.8 mmol/L	Population: No Outcomes: Yes Measurement: Yes Confounding: N/A Intervention: N/A

Predictors and Consequences of Severe Hypoglycemia in Adults with Diabetes – Systematic Review of the Evidence

Author Date Country Funding Source	Study Design Data Sources Length of Follow-up	Inclusion/Exclusion Criteria	Patient Characteristics	Intervention/ Control Target HbA1c	Definition of Severe Hypoglycemia	Study Quality
Liebl 2009[48] PREFER Europe 107 sites Industry	RCT 26 weeks	Inclusion criteria: Adults; BMI≤40; on 1 or 2 OHAs with or without insulin; HbA1c ≥ 7.0% and ≤ 12% Exclusion criteria: Cardiac disease, impaired hepatic or renal failure, proliferative retinopathy, recent treatment with 3 or more OHAs or use of short-acting or pre-mixed insulin in past 6 months	N=719 Age: 60 years % male: 57 BMI: 31 Type 2 (%): 100 HbA1c: 8.5%	Basal-bolus with insulin detemir and insulin aspart (N=541) Premixed analogue insulin with biphasic insulin aspart (n=178) target HbA1c not specified	Patient unable to treat themselves	Allocation concealment: Unclear Blinding: No Intention to treat analysis (ITT): No (1 dose) Withdrawals/dropouts adequately described: Yes
Lundkvist 2005[125] Sweden Industry	Cross-sectional Interviews of patients at primary care centers	Inclusion criteria: Age≥ 35; type 2 diabetes, treatment with OHA and/or insulin	N=309 115 w/ hypoglycemia; 194 without Age: 65 years Microvascular complication: 39% Macrovascular complication: 28%	NA	Required assistance of a third party to rectify the situation	Population: No Outcomes: No Measurement: No Confounding: Yes Intervention: N/A
Marre 2009[175] 21 countries 116 sites Industry	RCT 26 weeks	Inclusion criteria: Treated with OHAs for ≥ 3 months; 18–80 years old; HbA1c 7 —10%; BMI ≤ 45; Exclusion criteria: Insulin use within 3 months; impaired liver or renal function; uncontrolled HTN; cancer or any drugs apart from OHAs likely to affect glucose concentrations	N=1041 Age: 56 years % male: 50 Weight (lbs): 180.4 BMI: 30 Type 2 (%): 100 Duration of diabetes: 6.5 years HbA1c: 8.5%	**Glimepiride, 2-4mg/day PLUS:** a) Liraglutide 0.6 SC and rosiglitazone b) Liraglutide 1.2 SC and rosiglitazone c) Liraglutide 1.8 SC and rosiglitazone d) Liraglutide and rosiglitazone 4mg/day HbA1c<7%	Self-measured blood glucose = 3.0 mmol/l	Allocation concealment: Unclear Blinding: YesIntention to treat analysis (ITT): No (1 dose) Withdrawals/dropouts adequately described: Yes
Marre 2009[18] PREDICTIVE France Industry	Prospective Cohort Patient medical records 52 weeks	Inclusion criteria: Patients prescribed insulin detemir by physician, including those who switched from treatment with other basal insulin and insulin-naïve patients Exclusion criteria: Patients unlikely or unable to comply with the study protocol; patients not classified as diabetes type 1 or 2	N=1772 Type 1 diabetes (n=643) Type 2 diabetes (n=1129) Age: 57 years % male: 50 Weight (lb): 172.6 BMI: 28.2 Type 2 (%): 63.7 Duration of diabetes: 15.5 years Major hypoglycemia: 6.7% HbA1c: 8.6%	N/A	Severe CNS symptoms consistent with hypoglycemia; subject unable to treat himself/ herself and third-party intervention is needed; has one of the following: a) Blood glucose <2.8 mmol/l (50 mg/dl) b) Reversal of symptoms after food intake, glucagon or intravenous glucose	Population: No Outcomes: Yes Measurement: Yes Confounding: No Intervention: Yes

Predictors and Consequences of Severe Hypoglycemia in Adults with Diabetes – Systematic Review of the Evidence

Author Date Country Funding Source	Study Design Data Sources Length of Follow-up	Inclusion/Exclusion Criteria	Patient Characteristics	Intervention/ Control Target HbA1c	Definition of Severe Hypoglycemia	Study Quality
Marrett 2009;[81] Marrett 2011[87] United States Industry	Cross-sectional 2007 Health and Wellness Survey	Inclusion criteria: Those who reported being treated with one or more OHAAs any time during the previous 6 months Exclusion criteria: Patients who reported insulin use within the same previous 6 months	N=1984 Age: 58.1 % male: 56.7 BMI: 34.5 Duration of diabetes: 7.3 years Microvascular: 22.5% Heart attack: 8% Angina: 8.5% Stroke: 4.3% Peripheral Vascular Disease: 0.96% CHF: 4.3%	N/A	Required the assistance of others to manage symptoms or requiring medical assistance	Population: Yes Outcomes: Yes Measurement: No Confounding: No Intervention: N/A
Matthews 2010[49] Multinational Industry	RCT 2 years	Inclusion criteria: Men, non-fertile women and women of child-bearing potential using medically approved birth control; aged 18–73 years; Type 2 diabetes inadequately controlled (HbA1c 6.5–8.5%) by metformin monotherapy	N=3118 Age: 57.5 years % male: 53.5 Race/Ethnicity (%): White=86.8 Black=1.2 Asian=2.9 Hispanic=8.4 Other=0.7 Weight (lbs): 196.2 BMI: 31.8 Duration of diabetes: 5.7 HbA1c: 7.3% Current Smokers: 16.6%	Vidagliptin 50 bid Glimepiride starting at 2 mg Groups added to metformin therapy	Any episode requiring assistance of another party	Allocation concealment: No Blinding: Yes Intention to treat analysis (ITT): Yes Withdrawals/dropouts adequately described: No

Predictors and Consequences of Severe Hypoglycemia in Adults with Diabetes – Systematic Review of the Evidence

Author Date Country Funding Source	Study Design Data Sources Length of Follow-up	Inclusion/Exclusion Criteria	Patient Characteristics	Intervention/ Control Target HbA1c	Definition of Severe Hypoglycemia	Study Quality
Meneghini 2007[176] PREDICTIVE United States 1083 sites Industry	RCT 26 weeks	Inclusion criteria: Type 2 diabetes; ≥18 years old; HbA1c ≤12%; BMI ≤45; likely to benefit from initiation of detemir, addition of detemir to other therapy, change to detemir, or continuation of detemir Exclusion criteria: Any glucose lowering medication not indicated in combination with detemir; anticipate starting on another medication known to interfere with glucose metabolism (e.g., steroids); proliferative retinopathy or maculopathy; history of hypoglycemia unawareness or recurrent major hypoglycemia; pregnant; nursing; had serious illness	N=4937 Age: 59 years % male: 52 Race/Ethnicity (%): White=77 Black=17 Asian=2 Other=5 BMI: 33.8 Type 2 (%): 100 Duration of diabetes: 11.4 years HbA1c: 8.5%	Randomization by study site (n=1083) to: a) Intervention: self-adjustment of insulin according to algorithm b) Control: adjustment by investigator according to standard of care Everyone was on detemir qhs as basal insulin; other medications as needed No target HbA1c	Symptoms of low blood sugar that resolved with oral carbohydrates, glucagon or IV glucose AND blood sugar < 56 AND patient was unable to treat himself	Allocation concealment: Unclear Blinding: No Intention to treat analysis (ITT): No Withdrawals/dropouts adequately described: Yes
Miller 2001[100] United States Government	Cross Sectional Diabetes Clinic of the Grady Health System, Inc, Atlanta, Ga. April 1, 1999 – October 31, 1999	Inclusion criteria: Type 2 diabetes with follow-up data > 2 months	N=1055 Age: 60.9 years % male: 28.2 Race/Ethnicity (%): White=3.6 Black=93.8 Other=2.6 BMI: 33.0 Duration of diabetes: 10.8 years HbA1c: 7.6%	N/A	Loss of consciousness or other major alteration of mental status caused by hypoglycemia that required the assistance of another person to treat the condition	Population: Yes Outcomes: Yes Measurement: Yes Confounding: Yes Intervention: N/A
Moen 2009[75] United States Government/ Foundation	Retrospective cohort Veterans Health Administration fiscal year 2005 acute inpatient data files 12 months	Inclusion criteria: At least one acute care hospitalization between Oct 1, 2004 – Sept 30, 2005 and at least one outpatient measure of serum creatinine between week 1 and 1 year before hospitalization	N=243,222	N/A	Severity denoted by categorical glucose measures: ≥60 and <70 mg/dl; ≥50 and <60 mg/dl; <50 mg/dl	Population: Yes Outcomes: Yes Measurement: Yes Confounding: Yes Intervention: N/A

Author Date Country Funding Source	Study Design Data Sources Length of Follow-up	Inclusion/Exclusion Criteria	Patient Characteristics	Intervention/ Control Target HbA1c	Definition of Severe Hypoglycemia	Study Quality
Murata 2005[19] United States Government (VA)	Prospective cohort Mean: 41 weeks	Inclusion criteria: Type 2 taking at least 1 dose of long acting insulin daily; did not self-titrate insulin; stable for 2 months. Exclusion criteria: History of ETOH or SUD, chronic liver disease, pancreas insufficiency, chronic infectious disease, endocrinopathy, creatinine > 3, on corticosteroids or immunosuppressant drugs, insulin pump, life expectancy < 1 yr	N=344 Age: 66 years % male: 96 BMI: 32 Diabetes duration: 15 years Insulin treatment: 8 years Also on OHA: 48% HbA1c: 8.0%	N/A	Blood sugar< 60 with symptoms of affected mental function or requiring assistance of others	Population: Yes Outcomes: No Measurement: No Confounding: No Intervention: N/A
Nauck 2007;[177] **Seck 2010**[50] Multinational Industry	RCT 52 wks, then f/u for another year	Inclusion criteria: Age 18-78; Type 2 diabetes; not currently on an OHA or on an OHA other than metformin monotherapy at a dose ≥1500 mg/day or on metformin in combination with another OHA; HbA1c >6.5% and < 10%	N=1172 Age: 56.7 years % male: 59.2 Race/Ethnicity (%): White=73.9 Black=6.5 Hispanic=7.6 Asian=8.4 Other=3.6 Weight(lbs): 197.2 BMI: 31.3 Duration of diabetes: 6.4 years HbA1c: 7.7%	Sitagliptin 100mg qd Glipizide starting at 5 mg qd Groups added to metformin therapy	Required nonmedical assistance Required medical assistance	Allocation concealment: Unclear Blinding: Yes Intention to treat analysis (ITT): No Withdrawals/dropouts adequately described: Yes
Nauck 2009[53] **(LEAD-2)** 21 Countries, 170 sites Industry	RCT 26 weeks	Inclusion criteria: Type 2 diabetes; age 18-80 yrs; HbA1c 7-11% (if prestudy OHA monotherapy ≥3 months) or 7-10% (if prestudy combination OHA therapy ≥3 months); BMI ≤ 40 Exclusion criteria: Insulin use during previous 3 months	N=1087 Age: 57 years % male: 58 Race/Ethnicity (%): White=87 Black=3 Asian/Pacific Islander=9 Other=1 BMI: 31 Duration of diabetes: 7.6 years HbA1c: 8.4%	Liraglutide (once-daily) 1) 0.6 mg (n=242) 2) 1.2 mg (n=240) 3) 1.8 mg (n=242) Glimepiride (once-daily): 4 mg (n=242) Placebo (n=121)	Required third-party assistance	Allocation concealment: No Blinding: Yes (reported to be double-blind) Intention to treat analysis (ITT): No (excluded 4 who did not receive a treatment dose) Withdrawals/dropouts adequately described: Yes

Predictors and Consequences of Severe Hypoglycemia in Adults with Diabetes – Systematic Review of the Evidence

Author Date Country Funding Source	Study Design Data Sources Length of Follow-up	Inclusion/Exclusion Criteria	Patient Characteristics	Intervention/ Control Target HbA1c	Definition of Severe Hypoglycemia	Study Quality
Nichols 2010[26] United States Industry	Retrospective cohort database of patients newly started on insulin 49 months	Inclusion criteria: Type 2 diabetes, 18 or older with no prior insulin use who then were started on insulin between 1999-2004 Exclusion criteria: No HbA1c in the 6 months prior to insulin initiation or only had 1 insulin prescription filled	N=3332 Age: 60 years % male: 49 Duration of diabetes: 6.8 years BMI: 34 HbA1c: 9.3% Hypertension: 61% Current smokers: 12% CVD: 25% Nephropathy: 10% Retinopathy: 17%	N/A	Defined as ICD-9 251.0 and 251.2 during an outpatient visit	Population: Yes Outcomes: Yes Measurement: Yes Confounding: No Intervention: Yes
Olansky 2011[178] United States 229 sites Industry	RCT 44 weeks	Inclusion criteria: Type 2 diabetes; age 18-78; HbA1c ≥7.5% on diet; on no OHA for previous 4 months	N=815 Age: 49.7 years % male: 56.5 BMI: 33.4 Duration of diabetes: 3.4 years HbA1c: 9.9%	Sitagliptin 50/metformin 500 bid titrated up to 50/1000 bid (n=625) Metformin 500 bid titrated up to 1000 bid (N=621)	Required nonmedical or medical assistance	Allocation concealment: No Blinding: Yes Intention to treat analysis (ITT): No Withdrawals/dropouts adequately described: Yes
Panikar 2003[117] India NR	Prospective Cohort 6 months of triple drug therapy	Inclusion criteria: Duration of type 2 diabetes ≥ 5 years and being treated with insulin Exclusion criteria: Known renal failure or increased serum creatinine levels >1.5 mg/dl; cardiac abnormality-history of symptomatic angina, cardiac insufficiency or history of myocardial infarction or abnormal ECG; SGOT/SGPT more than two times upper limit of normal; more than 60 ml alcohol/ day	N=124 Age: 57.1 years % male: 47 Weight (lb): 149.7 Type 2 (%): 100 HbA1c: 11.5%	Triple drug combination of: pioglitazone 15 mg/d glibenclamide 5 mg metformin 500 mg three times a day Each in addition to insulin	"Significant hypoglycemia" Not defined in paper	Population: Yes Outcomes: Yes Measurement: No Confounding: No Intervention: Yes

Author Date Country Funding Source	Study Design Data Sources Length of Follow-up	Inclusion/Exclusion Criteria	Patient Characteristics	Intervention/ Control Target HbA1c	Definition of Severe Hypoglycemia	Study Quality
Pencek 2009[20] United States 116 sites Industry	Prospective cohort 6 months	Inclusion criteria: MDs selected patients they thought would benefit from pramlinitide	N=1297 Age: 48.7 years % male: 38.6 Race/Ethnicity (%): White=84.7 Black=9.6 Hispanic=3.8 Other=1.2 Weight (lbs): 214.6 BMI: 34.1 Duration of diabetes: 18.5 HbA1c: 8%	N/A	Patient reported as self-treatable or requiring assistance (either of another person (PASH) or of a medical (MASH))	Population: No Outcomes: Yes Measurement: No Confounding: No Intervention: N/A
Pettersson 2011[82] Sweden multicenter Industry	Cross-sectional Medical record review and self administered questionnaire	Inclusion criteria: Type 2 diabetes; age≥35; metformin and SU for at least 6 months Exclusion criteria: Type 1 diabetes; HIV or hepatitis; gestational diabetes; any treatment with insulin; any treatment with akarbos, repaglinid during last 6 months	N=430 Age: 69 years % male: 61 BMI: 28.7 Microvascular events: 20% Macrovascular events: 33% Major medical events: 23%	N/A	Severe: Needed the assistance of others to manage symptoms Very Severe: Needed medical attention	Population: Yes Outcomes: No Measurement: Yes Confounding: No Intervention: N/A
Pratley 2010[179] 11 European countries 158 sites Industry	RCT Open label 26 weeks	Inclusion criteria: Type 2 diabetes; age 18-80; HbA1c 7.5 - 10.0%; BMI < 45; metformin for at least 3 months Exclusion criteria: Treatment with any OHA except metformin within 3 months of trial; recurrent major hypoglycemia or hypoglycemic unawareness; present use of any drug except metformin that could affect glucose; impaired renal or hepatic function; clinically significant cardiovascular disease; or cancer	N=675 Age: 55.3 years % male: 52.9 Race/Ethnicity (%): White=86.6 Hispanic=16.2 Black=7.2 Asian Pacific Islander=2.0 Other=4.2 Weight (lbs): 206.4 BMI: 32.8 Duration of diabetes: 6.2 years HbA1c: 8.4%	Lirgulitide 1.2 mg qd (225) Lirgulitide 1.8 mg qd (221) Sitagliptin 100 mg qd (219)	Required third party assistance	Allocation concealment: Yes Blinding: No Intention to treat analysis (ITT): No Withdrawals/dropouts adequately described: Yes

**Predictors and Consequences of Severe Hypoglycemia
in Adults with Diabetes – Systematic Review of the Evidence**

Author Date Country Funding Source	Study Design Data Sources Length of Follow-up	Inclusion/Exclusion Criteria	Patient Characteristics	Intervention/ Control Target HbA1c	Definition of Severe Hypoglycemia	Study Quality
Quilliam 2011[27] United States Industry	Case-control Health care claims from the 2004 to 2008 MarketScan database (Ann Arbor, Michigan)	Inclusion criteria: Adults; 18+ years of age with at least 2 outpatient or inpatient claims for diabetes during 2004 to 2008 taking at least 1 OHA Exclusion criteria: At least 12 months of continuous eligibility within a non-capitated health plan after the initial fill date of an OHA, and those with 1 medical claim (inpatient or outpatient) for type 1 or gestational diabetes during the study period	N=14,729 Age: 54.8 years % male: 53.5	Cases: patients with hypoglycemic events (n=1339) Controls: patients without hypoglycemic events but with similar exposure status (n=13,390)	Requiring inpatient medical intervention	Population: Yes Outcomes: No Measurement: Yes Confounding: Yes Intervention: N/A
Quilliam 2011[183] United States Industry	Retrospective cohort Health care claims from the 2004 to 2008 MarketScan database	Inclusion criteria: Type 2 diabetes; age 18+; at least 2 claims for diabetes during study period; taking at least 1 OHA Exclusion criteria: At least 12 months continuous eligibility; 1 claim for type 1 or gestational diabetes	N=536,581 Age: 18-34 (3.3%) 35-49 (25.7%) 50-64 (70.8%) 65+ (0.1%) % male: 54% Insulin Use: 6.0% Macrovascular complications: 7.0% Microvascular complications: 4.3%	N/A	Required medical intervention	Population: Yes Outcomes: No Measurement: Yes Confounding: Yes Intervention: N/A

95

Author Date Country Funding Source	Study Design Data Sources Length of Follow-up	Inclusion/Exclusion Criteria	Patient Characteristics	Intervention/ Control Target HbA1c	Definition of Severe Hypoglycemia	Study Quality
Raskin 2009[31] United States 100 sites Industry	RCT 26 weeks	Inclusion criteria: Adults with type 2; currently on OHA medication monotherapy (at least 2 months) or dual therapy; HbA1c between 7.5 and 11% inclusive (monotherapy) or between 7.0 and 10% inclusive (dual therapy) Exclusion criteria: Pregnant or nursing women; significant disease history; any investigational drug within 4 weeks of screening; treatment with TZD or systemic corticosteroids within 2 months of screening; history of hypoglycemic unawareness or recurrent severe hyperglycemia	N=561	Repaglinide/metformin BID Repaglinide/metformin TID Rosiglitazone /metformin BID	Required the assistance of others	Allocation concealment: Unclear Blinding: No (open-label) Intention to treat analysis (ITT): No Withdrawals/dropouts adequately described: Yes
Rašlová 2004[112] 8 countries 31 sites Industry	Randomized, open-label trial 22 week treatment	Inclusion criteria: Men and women ≥18 years; BMI ≤40 kg/m²; HbA1c <12.0%; history of type 2 diabetes ≥1 year Exclusion criteria: Significant medical disorder; hypoglycemic unawareness or recurrent major hypoglycemia; pregnant or breast-feeding women; allergy to insulin	N=395 Age: 58.2 years % male: 42.1 Race/Ethnicity (%): Caucasian=99.7 Non-Caucasian=0.3 Weight (lbs): 177.7 BMI: 29.2 Type 2 (%): 100 Duration of diabetes: 14.1 years HbA1c: 8.1%	Insulin detemir (IDet) (100U/mL) in combo with insulin aspart (IAsp) (n=195) NPH insulin (NPH) (100IU/mL) in combo with regular human insulin (HIS) (n=199)	Individual unable to treat him/herself	Allocation Concealment: No Blinding: Yes- Intention to Treat Analysis (ITT): No Withdrawals/ Dropouts: Yes
Ratner 2002[34] United States 37 sites Industry	RCT 52 weeks	Inclusion criteria: Age 26-76; type 2 diabetes; on insulin for at least 6 months; HbA1c 7.5-13%, body weight +/-60% of desirable according to Met Life tables Exclusion criteria: IHD; uncontrolled HTN; GI or renal disease (CR > 2); unstable diabetic retinopathy; treatment with drugs known to affect gastric motility or glucose metabolism	N=538 Age: 56 years % male: 60 Race/Ethnicity (%): White=58 Black=9 Hispanic=7 Other=1 Unknown=25 BMI: 31 Duration of diabetes: 12 years HbA1c: 9.2%	Mealtime (tid) injections of placebo, or 30, 75, or 150 ug of pramlintide Target HbA1c < 8%	Events requiring assistance of another individual, or administration of glucagon, or IV glucose. Were then rated mild, moderate, severe by PI	Allocation Concealment: Unclear Blinding: Yes Intention to Treat Analysis (ITT): No (1 dose) Withdrawals/Dropouts adequately described: Yes

Predictors and Consequences of Severe Hypoglycemia in Adults with Diabetes – Systematic Review of the Evidence

Author Date Country Funding Source	Study Design Data Sources Length of Follow-up	Inclusion/Exclusion Criteria	Patient Characteristics	Intervention/ Control Target HbA1c	Definition of Severe Hypoglycemia	Study Quality
Rayman 2006[45] Multinational 90 sites Industry	RCT 26 weeks	Inclusion criteria: Age ≥ 18; Type 2 DM; > 6 months continuous insulin therapy; HbA1c 6.0 - 11.0%	N=890 Age: 60 years % male: 49.7 BMI: 31.3 Duration of diabetes: 13.5 years HbA1c: 7.5%	Insulin gluilsine and NPH (N=448) RHI + NPH (N=442)	Requiring assistance of another person and confirmed by blood sugar <36 mg/ dl or associated with prompt recovery with oral carbohydrate, IV glucose, or glucagon	Allocation concealment: Unclear Blinding: No (open-label) Intention to treat analysis (ITT): No Withdrawals/dropouts adequately described: Yes
Redelmeier 2009[129] Canada Government	Case control study Ontario Ministry of Transportation Medical Advisory Board	Inclusion criteria: Licensed drivers in Ontario 1/1/05-1/1/07 with commercial license annual review, report after crash, or diabetic patients reviewed for other reason Exclusion criteria: No HbA1c available	N=795 Age: 52 yr % male: 80 Duration of diabetes: approx 20 yrs HbA1c: ranged from 4.4-14.7%	N/A	Required outside assistance	Population: Yes Outcomes: Yes Measurement: No Confounding: Yes Intervention: N/A
Rhoads 2005[18] United States NR	Retrospective cohort MarketScan Health Productivity and Management Database (data from 5 large employers)	Inclusion criteria: Employees eligible in incur absence and/or short term disability with pharm. benefits; at least 12 mos continuous enrollment; at least 2 drug claims for same class of DM-related medications	N=442 with hypoglycemia Age: 44 years % male: 71	N/A	ICD-9-CM 250.8, 251.1, 251.2	Population: Yes Outcomes: Yes Measurement: Yes Confounding: Yes Intervention: N/A

Predictors and Consequences of Severe Hypoglycemia in Adults with Diabetes – Systematic Review of the Evidence

Author Date Country Funding Source	Study Design Data Sources Length of Follow-up	Inclusion/Exclusion Criteria	Patient Characteristics	Intervention/ Control Target HbA1c	Definition of Severe Hypoglycemia	Study Quality
Riddle 2003,[41] Dailey 2009,[132] INSULIN GLARGINE 4002 United States and Canada Industry	RCT 24 week	Inclusion criteria: Men and women; ages 30-70 years; diabetes for ≥ 2 years, treated with stable dose of 1 or 2 OHAs (sulfonylurea, metformin, pioglitazone, rosiglitazone) for ≥ 3 mos; BMI 26-40 kg/m²; HbA1c 7.5-10%; FPG ≥ 140 mg/dl at screening Exclusion criteria: Prior use of insulin except for gestational diabetes or for <1 wk; current use of α-glucosidase inhibitor or rapid-acting insulin secretagogue; use of other agents effecting glycemic control, history of ketoacidosis or self-reported inability to recognize hypoglycemia; serum alanine aminotransferase or aspratate aminotransferase > 2 times upper limit of normal	N=756 Age: 67 years % male: 56 Race/Ethnicity (%): White=84 Black=12 Asian=3 Multiracial=1 Hispanic=8 BMI: 32.4 Duration of diabetes: 8.7 years HbA1c: 8.6%	Glargine starting dose 10 IU at bedtime, titrated weekly NPH same HbA1c ≤7.0% was study outcome	Symptoms consistent with hypoglycemia during which the subject required the assistance of another person and was associated with either a glucose level <56mg/dl or prompt recovery after oral carbohydrate, intravenous glucose, or glucagon	Allocation concealment: Yes Blinding: No Intention-to-Treat Analysis (ITT): No (1 dose) Withdrawals/dropouts adequately described: Yes
Rosenstock 2008[189] Europe and United States 80 sites Industry	RCT 52 weeks	Inclusion criteria: Insulin naïve pts with type 2 diabetes; age ≥18; diabetes for at least 1 year; BMI < 40; HbA1c 7.5 – 10%; on one or two OHA for at least 4 months at least ½ the maximal recommended dose	N=582 Age: 58.9 years % male: 57.9 Race/Ethnicity (%): White=88.1 Black=5.8 Asian Pacific Islander=2.4 Other=3.6 Weight (lbs): 192.3 BMI: 30.5 Duration of diabetes: 9.1 years HbA1c: 8.6%	Detemir (291) Glargine (291) qhs titrated to target FPG <6.0	Required assistance from a third party	Allocation concealment: No Blinding: No Intention to treat analysis (ITT): Yes Withdrawals/dropouts adequately described: Yes

Predictors and Consequences of Severe Hypoglycemia in Adults with Diabetes – Systematic Review of the Evidence

Author Date Country Funding Source	Study Design Data Sources Length of Follow-up	Inclusion/Exclusion Criteria	Patient Characteristics	Intervention/ Control Target HbA1c	Definition of Severe Hypoglycemia	Study Quality
Rosenstock 2001[39] United States 59 sites Industry	RCT 28 weeks	Inclusion criteria: Type 2 diabetes, age 40-80, on insulin for ≥ 3 months HbA1c 7-12%, BMI < 40 Exclusion criteria: Significant hepatic or renal dysfunction, had received treatment with an OHA within prior 3 months	N=518 Age: 59 years % male: 60 Race/Ethnicity (%): White=80 Black=40 Hispanic=22 BMI: 30.6 Type 2 (%): 100 Duration of diabetes(years): 13.7 Duration of insulin use (years): 8.4 years Symptomatic hypoglycemia during screening:27% HbA1c: 8.6%	Glargine: qd NPH: qd or bid Target HbA1c: <6.7%	Event with symptoms consistent with hypoglycemia in which the subject required assistance of another person and was either accompanied by a blood glucose of < 2.0 mmol/L or had prompt recovery after oral carbohydrate, intravenous glucose, or glucagon administration	Allocation concealment: Unclear Blinding: No Intention to treat analysis (ITT): Yes Withdrawals/dropouts adequately described: Yes
Rosenstock 2009[35] United States and Canada Industry	RCT 5 years	Inclusion criteria: Age 30-70; Type 2 for ≥ 1 yr; stable dose for > 3months on OHAs or insulin alone or in combination; HbA1c 6-12% Exclusion criteria: Proliferative or severe non-proliferative retinopathy; history of laser vitrectomy or photocoagulation; use of insulin within 3 months; SBP >150 or DBP > 90; history of hypoglycemia unawareness	N=1024 Age: 55 years % male: 54 Weight (lbs): 217.8 BMI: 34 Type 2 (%): 100 Diabetes duration: 11 years Duration of insulin use (years): 5 years Renal insufficiency: 10% HbA1c: 8.4%	Insulin glargine (N=513) qd NPH insulin (N=504)bid	Symptomatic hypoglycemia requiring assistance and either with blood glucose levels of ≤3.1 mmol/l or treated with oral or injectable carbohydrate or glucagon injection	Allocation concealment: Unclear Blinding: No Intention to treat analysis (ITT): No (1 dose) Withdrawals/dropouts adequately described: Yes

Predictors and Consequences of Severe Hypoglycemia in Adults with Diabetes – Systematic Review of the Evidence

Author Date Country Funding Source	Study Design Data Sources Length of Follow-up	Inclusion/Exclusion Criteria	Patient Characteristics	Intervention/ Control Target HbA1c	Definition of Severe Hypoglycemia	Study Quality
Russell-Jones 2009[54] (LEAD-5 met+SU) 17 Countries, 107 sites Industry	RCT 26 weeks	Inclusion criteria: Type 2 diabetes; age 18-80; treated with OHAs for ≥3 months before screening; HbA1c 7.5-10% if on oral monotherapy or 7-10% if on combination therapy; BMI ≤45 Exclusion criteria: Insulin use within 3 months prior to trial; impaired hepatic or renal function; clinically significant CV disease; proliferative retinopathy or maculopathy; hypertension (≥180/100 mmHg) or cancer; pregnant; recurrent hypoglycemia or hypoglycemia unawareness; seropositive for hepatitis B antigen or hepatitis C antibody; using any other medications that could affect blood glucose levels	N=576 Age: 57.5 years % male: 56.6 Race/Ethnicity: NR Weight (kg): 85.3 BMI: 30.5 Duration of diabetes: 9.4 years HbA1c: 8.3%	Randomized if received glimepiride (4 mg) and metformin (2 g) for at least 3 weeks and had fasting glucose of 7.5 to 12.8 mmol/l after 6 week run-in Liraglutide once-daily (1.8 mg) (blinded) (n=230) Liraglutide placebo once-daily (blinded) (n=114) Insulin glargine once-daily (open label) (n=232) All in combination with metformain and glimepiride (open label)	Requiring third-party assistance	Allocation concealment: Yes Blinding: Partial, participants, investigators, study monitors for liraglutide and placebo groups (see interventions) Intention to treat analysis (ITT): No (excluded 5 who did not receive a treatment dose) Withdrawals/dropouts adequately described: Yes
Saloranta 2002[59] 12 Countries, 103 sites Industry	RCT 24 weeks	Inclusion criteria: Men and women, age 30 or older; type 2 diabetes for ≥6 weeks; maintained on diet alone for ≥6 weeks before screening; FPG 7.0-8.3 mmol/L Exclusion criteria: Type 1 diabetes; pancreatic injury; acute metabolic or significant diabetic complications	N=675 Age: 60.2 years % male: 62.5 Race/Ethnicity (%): Caucasian=95.6 Black=1 Asian=1.3 Other=2.1 BMI: 23.9 Duration of diabetes: 3.6 years HbA1c: 6.5%	Nateglinide 30, 60, or 120 mg (maintain diet and exercise during study) Goal HbA1c <6.0%	Requiring outside assistance	Allocation concealment: Unclear Blinding: Yes - double Intention to treat analysis (ITT): Unclear Withdrawals/dropouts adequately described: No
Sarkar 2010[78] United States Government	Cross-sectional Survey of patients from Kaiser Permanente northern California 62% Response Rate	Inclusion criteria: Type 2 diabetes on medications; age 30-75	N=14,357 Age: 58 years % male: 51 Race/Ethnicity (%): White=22 Black=17 Latino=23 Asian=20 Other/mixed=20 Duration of diabetes: 10 years HbA1c: 7.6%	N/A	Participant report of having a "severe low blood sugar reaction, such as passing out or needing help to treat the reaction"	Population: Yes Outcomes: Yes Measurement: No Confounding: Yes Intervention: N/A

Predictors and Consequences of Severe Hypoglycemia in Adults with Diabetes – Systematic Review of the Evidence

Author Date Country Funding Source	Study Design Data Sources Length of Follow-up	Inclusion/Exclusion Criteria	Patient Characteristics	Intervention/Control Target HbA1c	Definition of Severe Hypoglycemia	Study Quality
Sato 2010[106] Japan NR	Case-control Seirei Hamamatsu General Hospital January 2005 – October 2009	Inclusion criteria: Type 2 diabetes treated with sulfonylurea Exclusion criteria: Patients with factitious hypoglycemia owing to the mistaken use of medicine or attempted suicide, severe acute infection, heart failure, acute coronary syndrome, hepatic dysfunction, endocrine disorders, or renal failure	N=157 Age: 66 years % male: 59.9 BMI: 24 Duration of diabetes: 8.9 years HbA1c: 7.8%	Case: Admission to hospital with severe hypoglycemia (n=32) Control: Outpatients without severe hypoglycemia (n=125)	Characteristic symptoms and a plasma glucose level of less than 50 mg/dl which required intravenous glucose administration	Population: No Outcomes: No Measurement: No Confounding: No Intervention: N/A
Schernthaner 2004[57] Europe Industry	RCT 27 weeks	Inclusion criteria: Type 2 diabetes, >35 years old, treated for at least 3 months with diet alone or in combination with metformin or an α-glucosidase inhibitor HbA1c 6·9-11·5%, able to perform home blood glucose monitoring Exclusion criteria: Contraindication to study drugs, no effective contraception in women with child-bearing potential, elevated transaminases more than threefold the upper normal range	N=845 Age: 60.5 years % male: 51.5 Weight (lbs): 183.6 BMI: 30.6 Duration of diabetes: 5.7 years HbA1c: 8.3% Macrovascular: 21.4% Microvascular: 10.5%	Gliclazide modified release (MR) Glimepiride Both arms either as monotherapy or with pts current therapy maintained at a stable dose	Symptomatic episodes requiring external assistance owing to severe impairment in consciousness or behavior, with BGL < 3 mmol/L	Allocation concealment: Unclear Blinding: Yes Intention to treat analysis (ITT): No (1 dose) Withdrawals/dropouts adequately described: Yes
Shen 2008[101] United States NR	Cross-sectional National Inpatient Sample database	Inclusion criteria: Discharge diagnosis of diabetes Exclusion criteria: Age < 18, pregnancy, skin diagnoses, transfers to other hospitals, discharges with "missing values"	N=787,836 Age: 66 years % male: 46	N/A	"Acute hypoglycemic condition" as a discharge diagnosis	Population: Yes Outcomes: Yes Measurement: Yes Confounding: Yes Intervention: N/A
Shorr 1997[97] United States Government	Retrospective Cohort Tennessee Medicaid enrollees January 1, 1985, through December 31, 1989	Inclusion criteria: All Tennessee Medicaid enrollees aged 65 years and older who used insulin or oral hypoglycemic drugs from 1985 through 1989 and experienced severe hypoglycemia; 1 full year of Medicaid enrollment was required	N=586 Age: 78 years % male: 18 Race/Ethnicity (%): White=48 Non-white=52	N/A	Neuroglycopenic or autonomic symptoms, with a concomitant blood glucose determination of <50 mg/dL)	Population: Yes Outcomes: Yes Measurement: Yes Confounding: Yes Intervention: N/A

Predictors and Consequences of Severe Hypoglycemia in Adults with Diabetes – Systematic Review of the Evidence

Author Date Country Funding Source	Study Design Data Sources Length of Follow-up	Inclusion/Exclusion Criteria	Patient Characteristics	Intervention/ Control Target HbA1c	Definition of Severe Hypoglycemia	Study Quality
Sotiropoulos 2005[108] Greece NR	Case series Clinical records at a single hospital	Inclusion criteria: Patients admitted due to severe hypoglycemia	N=207 Age: 62 years % male: 41 Duration of diabetes: 7.4 years HbA1c: 6.8%	N/A	Comatose or pre-comatose on arrival at ED; glucose < 50, and needing IV glucose	Population: Yes Outcomes: Yes Measurement: No Confounding: Yes Intervention: N/A
Stahl 1999[28] Switzerland NR	Case series Medical records for ER admissions at the University Hospital, Basle Switzerland 12 years	Inclusion criteria: Type 2 diabetes treated with long versus short-acting sulfonylurea Exclusion criteria: Insulin treatment	N=28 Age: 71.8 years % male: 46.4 Duration of diabetes: 10.2 years	Long- acting sulfonylurea (n=16) Short-acting sulfonylurea (n=12)	Episodes of hypoglycemia leading to hospital admission	Population: No Outcomes: Yes Measurement: No Confounding: Yes Intervention: Yes
Standl 2006[180] 11 European countries, 113 centers Industry	RCT 24 weeks	Inclusion criteria: men or women, age 18-80 years, type 2 diabetes diagnosed at least 3 years prior to study entry, on oral anti-diabetics for at least 6 months with poor control (HbA1c ≥7.5% and ≤10.5%, FBG ≥120 mg/dl), BMI ≤35 kg/m²	N=624 Age: 61.8 years % male: 54.5 BMI: 28.5 Type 2 (%): 100 Duration of diabetes: 9.9 years HbA1c: 8.8%	AM Glargine titrated to target FBG ≤ 100 mg/dl and AM glimepiride (6 to 9 am) PM Glargine n=312; titrated to target FBG ≤ 100 mg/dl and AM glimepiride (6 to 9 am)	Symptoms consistent with hypoglycemia during which the person required the assistance of another person and was associated with a blood glucose level <50 mg/dl or with prompt recovery after oral carbohydrate, IV glucose or glucagon administration	Allocation concealment: Unclear Blinding: No Intention to treat analysis (ITT): No Withdrawals/dropout adequately described: No
Stepka 1993[98] Poland NR	Retrospective Cohort Medical records from GI and Metabolic Diseases of one hospital, 1975 - 1989	Inclusion criteria: Diabetic patients admitted for serious hypoglycemia	N=137 Age: 66.4 years Type 2: 73.7% Treated with insulin: 26.3%	N/A	Requiring immediate aid in a health care institution	Population: Yes Outcomes: Yes Measurement: No Confounding: Yes Intervention: N/A

Predictors and Consequences of Severe Hypoglycemia in Adults with Diabetes – Systematic Review of the Evidence

Author Date Country Funding Source	Study Design Data Sources Length of Follow-up	Inclusion/Exclusion Criteria	Patient Characteristics	Intervention/ Control Target HbA1c	Definition of Severe Hypoglycemia	Study Quality
Stork 2007[130] Netherlands Foundation	Case Control University Medical Center Utrecht, Netherlands	Inclusion criteria: Adults ages 20 to 65 with a diabetes duration of 2 years, absence of cardiovascular disease or neuropathy, visual acuity > 16/20 in both eyes, drivers license Exclusion criteria: Medication use that would influence hypoglycemia counter-regulation.	N=20 (Type 2 diabetes) Age: 51.6 years % male: 80 Weight (lbs): 196.7 BMI: 28.3 Duration of diabetes: 8.7 years HbA1c: 7.9%	Type 1 diabetes with impaired hypoglycemic awareness Type 1 diabetes with normal hypoglycemic awareness Type 2 diabetes with normal awareness	N/A	Population: No Outcomes: Yes Measurement: No Confounding: No Intervention: Yes
Sugarman 1991[96] United States NR	Retrospective Cohort Medical records for all hospital discharges from Navajo Area Indian Health Service facilities October 1st 1983 to September 30th 1988	Exclusion criteria: Children, intentional drug overdose, non-diabetic	113 diabetic patients with 130 admissions (126 admissions among 109 patients who had been prescribed hypoglycemic agents) Race/ethnicity: Native American (100%) Duration of diabetes: 11.9 years (based on data from 108 patients)	N/A	Definition not given - all patients had been admitted to a hospital	Population: Yes Outcomes: Yes Measurement: Yes Confounding: No Intervention: N/A
UK Hypoglycaemia Study Group (UKHSG) 2007[190] United Kingdom 6 centers Government	Prospective cohort study 9–12 months	Inclusion criteria: Type 2 diabetes; patients with type 1 diabetes for < 5 years or > 15 years. Exclusion criteria: HbA1c >9%, measured centrally by an HPLC; severe diabetic complications, e.g., binocular visual acuity <6/12, major amputation, severe peripheral sensory neuropathy; treatment with metformin or acarbose alone; seizures unrelated to hypoglycemia; concurrent malignant disease; severe systemic diseases unrelated to diabetes; pregnancy Insulin users had to be taking two or more injections daily	N=274 Age: 57.2 years % male: 68.2 BMI: 29.8 Type 2 (%): 43 HbA1c: 7.5%	Subjects were given hypoglycemia reporting forms, on which they were asked to document the time, duration, symptoms, glucose level (if checked) and treatment required during any episode of hypoglycemia	Requiring help for recovery	Population: Yes Outcomes: No Measurement: No Confounding: No Intervention: N/A

Author Date Country Funding Source	Study Design Data Sources Length of Follow-up	Inclusion/Exclusion Criteria	Patient Characteristics	Intervention/ Control Target HbA1c	Definition of Severe Hypoglycemia	Study Quality
UKPDS 33 1998[21] United Kingdom 23 sites Government/ Foundation/ Industry	RCT Median: 11 years	Inclusion criteria: Newly diagnosed with diabetes (confirmed with FPG > 6mmol/l); age 25 to 65 years Exclusion criteria: Ketouria > 3 mmol/l; myocardial infarction in the previous year; current angina or HF; >1 major vascular episode;, serum creatinine > 175 umol/l; retinopathy requiring photocoagulation; malignant hypertension; uncorrected endocrine abnormality; occupation precluding insulin therapy; severe concurrent illness; inadequate comprehension	N=3867 Age: 59 years % male: 59 Race/Ethnicity (%): Caucasian=78 Afro-Caribbean=12 Asian=10 Weight (lbs): 178.2 BMI: 29.1 Type 2 (%): 100 HbA1c: 7.3%	FPG goal of 6 mmol/L. (n=2729); these patients received dietary advice; sulfonylureas used were: chlorpropamide 100-500mg; glibenclamide 2.5-20mg; glipizide 2.5-40mg. FPG goal of15 mmol/L. (n=1138)	Requiring third-party assistance or hospitalization	Allocation Concealment: Yes Blinding: Unclear Intention to Treat Analysis (ITT): Yes Withdrawals/dropouts adequately described: Unclear
UKPDS 34 1998[29] United Kingdom 23 sites Government/ Foundation/ Industry	RCT 10 years	Inclusion criteria: Newly diagnosed with diabetes (confirmed with FPG > 6mmol/l); age 25 to 65 years Exclusion criteria: Ketouria > 3 mmol/l; myocardial infarction in the previous year; current angina or HF; >1 major vascular episode; serum creatinine > 175 umol/l; retinopathy requiring photocoagulation; malignant hypertension; uncorrected endocrine abnormality; occupation precluding insulin therapy; severe concurrent illness; inadequate comprehension	N=743 Age: 59 years % male: 59 Race/Ethnicity (%): White=78 Afro-Caribbean=12 Asian=10 Weight (lbs): 178.2 BMI: 29.1 Type 2 (%): 100 HbA1c: 7.3%	Of 1704 overweight pts 743 were randomized: Diet (N=411) Intense glucose control (w/ metformin) (N=342)	Required third party help or medical intervention	Allocation Concealment: Yes Blinding: Unclear Intention to Treat Analysis (ITT): Yes Withdrawals/dropouts adequately described: Unclear
Valensi 2009[22] IMPROVE 11 countries Industry	Prospective Cohort N/A	Inclusion criteria: Type 2 dm newly started on BIASP30/70	N=52,419 Age: 55 years % maie: 57 Weight (%): 156.2 BMI: 26 Duration of diabetes: 7 years HbA1c: 9.3%	N/A	Severe CNS symptoms; patient unable to self-treat; accompanied by blood sugar < 50 or symptoms reversed after carbohydrate intake, glucagon or IV glucose	Population: Yes Outcomes: No Measurement: No Confounding: No Intervention: N/A

104

Predictors and Consequences of Severe Hypoglycemia in Adults with Diabetes – Systematic Review of the Evidence

Author Date Country Funding Source	Study Design Data Sources Length of Follow-up	Inclusion/Exclusion Criteria	Patient Characteristics	Intervention/ Control Target HbA1c	Definition of Severe Hypoglycemia	Study Quality
Vexiau, 2008[126] France 98 primary care clinics Industry	Cross-sectional Survey of MDs and patients	Inclusion criteria: ≥ 35 years old, type 2, on SU and metformin for at least 6 months Exclusion criteria: Using insulin, type 1, being treated for hepatitis or HIV, h/o gestational diabetes	N=400 Age: 62 years % male: 53 Weight (lbs): 178.2 Duration of diabetes > 7 years: 46% Current smoking: 14% HbA1c: 7.2%		Severe-needing third party assistance Very severe-needing medical attention	Population: No Outcomes: No Measurement: No Confounding: Yes Intervention: N/A
Weir, 2011[147] Canada Government	Case-control Ontario Health Administrative database January 2002 – March 2008	Inclusion criteria: Outpatients 66 years and older; diabetes mellitus; prescriptions for glyburide, insulin or metformin	N=2650	Normal renal function: Case (N=204) Control (N=802) Impaired renal function: Case (N=354) Control (N=1290)	Presenting to the hospital or emergency room with an admission diagnosis of hypoglycemia	Population: No Outcomes: No Measurement: Yes Confounding: No Intervention: N/A
Whitmer, 2009[94] United States Government	Cohort Registry data from Kaiser Permanente (KP) N/A	Inclusion criteria: Enrollees in KP as of January 2003; no prior diagnosis of dementia, MCI, or memory loss; history of type 2 diabetes; age ≥ 55 years old	N=16,667 Age: 65 years % male: 55 Race/Ethnicity (%): White=63 Black=11 Hispanic=11 Asian=12 Duration of diabetes: 9.6 years At least 1 episode of hypoglycemia: 8.8% HbA1c: 8.1%	NA	Hospitalization and ED codes for hypoglycemia before 2003	Population: Yes Outcomes: Yes Measurement: Yes Confounding: Yes Intervention: N/A

Author Date Country Funding Source	Study Design Data Sources Length of Follow-up	Inclusion/Exclusion Criteria	Patient Characteristics	Intervention/ Control Target HbA1c	Definition of Severe Hypoglycemia	Study Quality
Williams-Herman, 2009[113] 18 countries 140 sites Industry	RCT 54 weeks	Inclusion criteria: 18-78years old; not on an OHA; HbA1c ≥7.5% to ≤ 11% after a run-in period w/ no meds; good compliance during second placebo run in period	N=1091 Age: 53.5 % male: 57 BMI: 32 Duration of diabetes: 4 years HbA1c: 8.5%	a) Metformin 1000 mg bid (n=78) b) Sitagliptin 100 mg qd (n=106) c) Metformin 500 mg bid (n=122) d) Metformin 1000 mg bid (n=137) e) Sitagliptin 50 bid + metformin 500 bid (n=148) f) Sitagliptin 50 bid +metformin 100mg bid (n=157)	Requiring medical intervention or exhibiting markedly depressed level of consciousness, including loss of consciousness, or seizure	Allocation concealment: Unclear Blinding: Yes Intention to treat analysis (ITT): No Withdrawals/dropouts adequately described: Yes
Zargar, 2009[131] India NR	Retrospective Cohort Hospital records of admissions to Sher-i-Kashmir Institute of Medical Sciences 9 years	Inclusion criteria: Death certificate mentioning diabetes as underlying or contributory factor	N=741 Age: 58.8 years	N/A Target HbA1c< 7%	Hypoglycemia noted as a cause of, or contributing cause of death	Population: No Outcomes: Yes Measurement: No Confounding: Yes Intervention: N/A
Zinman, 2009[182] United States and Canada 96 sites Industry	RCT 26 weeks	Inclusion criteria: 18-80 years old; HbA1c 7-11% on pre-study OHA for ≥ 3 months; BMI ≤ 45 Exclusion criteria: Use of insulin during previous 3 months	N=533 Age: 55 years % male: 57 Race/Ethnicity (%): White=82 Black=12 Asian=2 Hispanic=15 Other=3 BMI: 33 Type 2 (%):100 Duration of diabetes: 9 years HbA1c: 8.5%	Group 1 (n= 178) 1.2 mg ligragulatide qd sc Group 2 (178) 1.8 mg lig qd sc Group 3 (n=177) placebo PLUS metformin and rosiglitazone in all 3 groups	Requiring third party assistance or medical intervention	Allocation concealment: Yes Blinding: Yes Intention to treat analysis (ITT): Yes Withdrawals/dropouts adequately described: Yes

AE = Adverse Event; BMI = Body Mass Index; CABG = Coronary Artery Bypass Grafting; CHF = Congestive Heart Failure; CK = Creatinine Kinase; CNS = Central Nervous System; CV = Cardiovascular; CVA = Cerebrovascular Accident; d/c = Discontinued; ER = Emergency Room; ESRD = End-stage Renal Disease; ETOH = Alcohol; GI = Gastrointestinal; GP = General Practitioner; HbA1c = Hemoglobin A1c; HTN = Hypertension; LVH = Left Ventricular Hypertrophy; MI = Myocardial Infarction; N/A = Not Applicable; NR = Not Reported; OHA = Oral Hypoglycemic Agent; RCT = Randomized Controlled Trial; SMBG = Self-monitored Blood Glucose; SU = Sulfonylurea; SUD = Substance Use Disorder; TZD = Thiazolidinedione; SU = Sulfonylurea

Table 2. Characteristics of Studies Included in Extended Analysis for Key Question #1

Author/Year/ Country/ Funding Source	Study Design Data sources Length of Follow-up	Population	Definition of Hypoglycemia	Results	Study Quality
Alvarez-Guisasola, 2008[85] 7 European countries Industry	Cross-sectional Questionnaire	N=1709 Type 2, age > 30, who had had a SU or TZD added to metformin in the previous 5 years	Self-report of episodes in past year, rated: 1. no interruption in activities 2. interrupt in activities but no help required 3. needed assistance of others 4. needed medical attention	38% reported one or more episodes of any severity; 26.8% reported level 3 and 5.1% reported level 4	Population: Yes Outcomes: No Measurement: No Confounding: Yes Intervention: N/A
Akram, 2006[34] Denmark Danish MRC and industry	Cross-sectional Questionnaire	N=401 of 671 asked to participate Type 2, exclusions: on SUs, on dialysis, concomitant malignancy, pregnancy, inability to complete questionnaire	Severe: required assistance of another person	66/401 (16.5%) had at least one severe event in the past year	Population: No Outcomes: Yes Measurement: No Confounding: Yes Intervention: N/A
Chan, 2010[73] China, Taiwan, Malaysia, Thailand Industry	Cross-sectional Questionnaire	N=2257 Type 2, older than 30, on OHA for at least 6 months	Self-report of episodes in past 6 months, rated: 1. no interruption in activities 2. interrupt in activities but no help required 3. needed assistance of others 4. needed medical attention	66 + 94 (160) of 2257 reported one or more severe or very severe events (7%)	Population: No Outcomes: Yes Measurement: No Confounding: No Intervention: N/A
Donnelly, 2005[72] Scotland Industry	Prospective cohort	267 Type 1 and 2 (N=173)	Required 3d party assistance, self report by diary	5 type 2 patients had one or more severe events over 1 month (5/173=2.8%)	Population: No Outcomes: No Measurement: Yes Confounding: Yes Intervention: N/A
Henderson, 2003[76] Edinburgh Government	Cross-sectional Questionnaire	N=215 type 2 diabetics treated with insulin at one clinic	Required external assistance; approx estimates of number of episodes in past year	32 (15%) people reported one or more severe episodes in past year	Population: No Outcomes: Yes Measurement: No Confounding: No Intervention: N/A
Honkasalo, 2010[77] Finland Foundation	Cross-sectional Questionnaire, EMRs, ambulance records	N=680 Patients over age 18 with Type 1 or Type 2 DM (n=480) all on insulin living in two communities	Needs the help of another person to recover	53/480 T2DM patients (12.3%) had one or more severe (self reported) episodes over 1 year; 10/53 required ambulance or emergency care	Population: No Outcomes: Yes Measurement: No Confounding: No Intervention: N/A

Predictors and Consequences of Severe Hypoglycemia in Adults with Diabetes – Systematic Review of the Evidence

Author/Year/ Country/ Funding Source	Study Design Data sources Length of Follow-up	Population	Definition of Hypoglycemia	Results	Study Quality
Jennings, 1989[80] England Industry	Cross-sectional Questionnaire	N=219 Age 40-65 with type 2 attending a single clinic who were treated with OHAs	Symptoms associated with a blood sugar reading of < 3 mmol and precipitated by reduced carbohydrate intake or increased exertion; relieved by carbohydrates; occurred after the institution of OHA therapy; and no other explanation for the hypoglycemic episode	In past 6 months: 41/203 (20%) patients on SU; 0/16 patients on metformin	Population: No Outcomes: Yes Measurement: No Confounding: No Intervention: N/A
Lecomte, 2008[79] France NR	Cross-sectional Claims data and survey of patients and providers	Random sample of 10,000 adults (36% responded) Treated for diabetes and living in France sent a questionnaire	Required the help of another person	26.5 % of 635 T2D on insulin and 6.3% of 2689 T2DM on OHA reported one or more severe episode in 2001	Population: No Outcomes: Yes Measurement: No Confounding: No Intervention: N/A
Lee, 2010[88] United States Industry	Retrospective cohort Administrative claims data	400 on NPH and 1698 on glargine T2DM patients < 65 years old, NOT pregnant, and were in the database for 6 months pre and 6 months post index date; index date was first prescribed for glargine or NPH	ICD 9 codes 251.0x, 251.1x, 251.2x, 250.3x. A hypoglycemic-related hospitalization event was defined by at least one claim with the codes above during a hospitalization	NONE in either group	Population: Yes Outcomes: No Measurement: Yes Confounding: Yes Intervention: N/A
Marrett, 2011[87] United States Industry	Population based survey	N=1984 Type 2 diabetes treated with one or more OHA in past 6 months but NOT on insulin	Severe—needed assistance of others Very severe—needed medical assistance	In past 6 months , 13% reported severe and 4% reported very severe episodes	Population: Yes Outcomes: Yes Measurement: No Confounding: Yes Intervention: N/A
Moen, 2009[81] United States Government	Retrospective cohort	N=243,222 VHA database of patients with CKD who had a t least one hospitalization in 2004-2005 and at least one outpatient measurement of CR between 1week and 1 year before they were hospitalized	Among 92,003 CKD patients with diabetes, 9264 had at least one glucose < 50 in the database		Population: Yes Outcomes: Yes Measurement: Yes Confounding: Yes Intervention: N/A
Neil, 2007[74] United States Government (VA)	Patient survey	N=11,529 Type 2 diabetics on SU but not insulin	Required assistance of another person	5965 responses to this question 538/5965 (9%) identified the episode as severe	Population: Yes Outcomes: Yes Measurement: No Confounding: Yes Intervention: Yes

Predictors and Consequences of Severe Hypoglycemia in Adults with Diabetes – Systematic Review of the Evidence

Author/Year/ Country/ Funding Source	Study Design Data sources Length of Follow-up	Population	Definition of Hypoglycemia	Results	Study Quality
Pettersson, 2011[82] Sweden (multicenter) Industry	Cross-sectional Patient survey	N=430 Patients with type 2 dm, age 35 or older, on metformin and SU for past 6 months	1. Mild: no interruption in activities 2. Moderate: interrupt in activities but no help required 3. Severe: needed assistance of others 4. Very severe: needed medical attention.	17% reported level 2; 1% reported level 3 and 1% reported level 4 hypoglycemic episode within past 6 months	Population: No Outcomes: Yes Measurement: No Confounding: No Intervention: N/A
Sarkar, 2010[73] United States Government	Cross-sectional patient survey linked with medical records	N=14,357 Adults with type 2 diabetes treated with OHAs past year	Survey question: In the past year, how many times have you had SEVERE low blood sugar reaction such as passing out or needing help to the treat the reaction?	1579 (11%) reported at least one episode; Insulin: 59% Mixed OHAs 23% Secretagogues alone: 13% Metformin alone: 5% 129/1579 (8%) had evidence of a documented ER visit or hospitalization for hypoglycemia in the prior year	Population: Yes Outcomes: Yes Measurement: No Confounding: Yes Intervention: N/A
Stargardt, 2009[83] Germany 92 clinics Industry	Patient survey	N=392 Type 2, 35 years old or older, treated in prior 6 months with either a combination of metformin and a glitazone or met and a SU	1. No interruption in activities 2. interrupt in activities but no help required 3. needed assistance of others 4. needed medical attention.	w/in previous 6 months 9/392 reported severe (#3) and 6/392 reported very severe (#4)	Population: No Outcomes: No Measurement: No Confounding: No Intervention: N/A
Williams, 2011[86] United States Industry	Cross-sectional Patient survey	N=10374 Patients with T2DM currently on one or more OHAs but not insulin invited….of whom **2074** completed the survey	If you answered yes to: In the prior 2 weeks did you have either "symptoms of low blood sugar" or "low blood sugar in the middle of the night" some most or all of the time	286/2074 (14%)	Population: Yes Outcomes: Yes Measurement: No Confounding: Yes Intervention: N/A

CKD = Chronic Kidney Disease; EMRs = Electronic Medical Records; ER = Emergency Room; HbA1c = Hemoglobin A1c; N/A = Not Applicable; NR = Not Reported; OHA = Oral Hypoglycemic Agent; RCT = Randomized Controlled Trial; SU = Sulfonylurea; T2DM = Type 2 diabetes mellitus; TZD = Thiazolidinedione; SU = Sulfonylurea

Table 3. Incidence of Severe Hypoglycemia by Treatment Arms

Table 3a. Intensive versus Standard Glycemic Control Studies

Study and year	Study type	Study duration	Intervention Control	Hypoglycemia Incidence % (n/N)	Risk ratio [95% CI]
Duckworth (VADT) 2009[5]	RCT	5.6 yrs	Intensive control	8.5 (76/892)	2.74 [1.79 to 4.18]
			Standard control	3.1 (28/899)	
ACCORD 2008[3]	RCT	3.5 yrs	Intensive control	16.6 (849/5128)	3.10 [2.72 to 3.53]
			Standard control	5.3 (274/5123)	
ADVANCE 2008[4]	RCT	5 yrs	Intensive control	2.7 (150/5571)	1.88 [1.44 to 2.46]
			Standard control	1.5 (81/5669)	
UKPDS 33 1998*[21]	RCT	10 yrs	Intensive control	1.1 (33/3071)	1.53 [0.71 to 3.30]
			Standard control	0.7 (8/1138)	
Abraira (VA-CSDM) 1995[30]	RCT	2.3 yrs	Intensive control	6.7 (5/75)	2.60 [0.52 to 12.99]
			Standard control	2.6 (2/78)	
		Totals	Intensive control	7.6 (1113/14737)	2.40 [1.76 to 3.27]
			Standard control	3.0 (393/12907)	

*Data obtained from Hemmingsen B, Lund SS, Gluud C, Vaag A, Almdal T, Hemmingsen C, Wetterslev J. Targeting intensive glycaemic control versus targeting conventional glycaemic control for type 2 diabetes mellitus. *Cochrane Database of Systematic Reviews* 2011, Issue 6. Art. No.: CD008143. DOI: 10.1002/14651858.CD008143.pub2.

Table 3b. Insulin Studies

Study and year	Study type	Study duration	Intervention(s) Control	Hypoglycemia Incidence % (n/N)
A. Regular insulin and Lispro studies: fast-short acting				
Anderson, 1997[47] (crossover study)	RCT	26 wks	Regular human insulin phase	0.6 (4/722)
			Insulin lispro phase	0.1 (1/722)
B. Insulin aspart studies: rapid-acting				
Holman, 2009[43] (4T study)	RCT	3 yrs	Prandial insulin aspart	2.1 (5/239)
			Biphasic insulin aspart	2.6 (6/235)
			Insulin detemir (basal)	0.9 (2/234)
C. Biphasic insulin: intermediate- and fast-acting mixture				
Berntorp, 2011[15]	Prospective cohort	26 wks	Biphasic insulin aspart	0.2 (2/1154)
Buse, 2011[36]	RCT	2.5 yrs	Insulin lispro 75/25 mix	4.2 (20/473)
			Insulin glargine (long-acting)	2.9 (12/419)
Holman 2009[43] (4T study)	RCT	3 yrs	Biphasic insulin aspart	2.6 (6/235)
			Prandial insulin aspart	2.1 (5/239)
			Insulin detemir (basal)	0.9 (2/234)
Liebl, 2009[48]	RCT		Biphasic insulin aspart	0/178
			Insulin detemir and insulin aspart	0.9 (5/537)
Valensi (IMPROVE) 2009[22]	Prospective cohort	26 wks	Biphasic insulin aspart	0.13 (69/52,419) 0.008 events per patient-year
D. Mixed fast and long-acting insulins studies				
Liebl, 2009[48]	RCT	26 wks	Insulin detemir and insulin aspart	0.9 (5/537)
			Biphasic insulin aspart	0/178
Rayman, 2006[45]	RCT	26 wks	Regular human insulin + NPH	1.6 (7/442)
			Insulin glulisine + NPH	0.5 (2/448)
Dailey, 2004[46]	RCT	26 wks	Regular human insulin + NPH	1.2 (5/441)
			Insulin glulisine + NPH	1.4 (6/435)
E. NPH insulin studies: intermediate acting				

Study and year	Study type	Study duration	Intervention(s) Control	Hypoglycemia Incidence % (n/N)
Rosenstock, 2009[35]	RCT	5 yrs	NPH insulin	11.1 (55/504)
			Insulin glargine	7.6 (38/513)
Rayman, 2007[45]	RCT	26 wks	NPH (basal therapy) + regular human insulin	1.6 (7/442)
			NPH (basal therapy) + insulin glulisine	0.5 (2/448)
Haak, 2005[33]	RCT	26 wks	Insulin detemir	<2% both arms (numbers not given)
			NPH insulin	
Dailey, 2004[46]	RCT	26 wks	NPH (basal therapy) + regular human insulin	1.2 (5/441)
			NPH (basal therapy) + insulin glulisine	1.4 (6/435)
Fritsche, 2003[44]	RCT	24 wks	NPH insulin + glimepiride (G) 3 mg	2.6 (6/232)
			Bedtime Insulin glargine + G	1.8 (4/227)
			Morning Insulin glargine + G	2.1 (5/236)
Riddle, 2003[41]	RCT	24 wks	Adjunct NPH insulin to 1-2 oral antiglycemic agents (sulfonylurea, metformin, or glitazone)	1.8 (7/389)
			Adjunct Insulin glargine to 1-2 oral antiglycemic agents (sulfonylurea, metformin, or glitazone)	2.5 (9/367)
Rosenstock, 2001[39]	RCT	28 wks	NPH insulin	2.3 (6/259)
			Insulin glargine	0.4 (1/259)
F. Insulin detemir studies: long-acting				
Holman, 2009 (4T study)[43]	RCT	3 yrs	Insulin detemir (basal)	0.9 (2/234)
			Insulin aspart (prandial)	2.1 (5/239)
			Biphasic insulin aspart	2.6 (6/235)
Liebl, 2009[48]	RCT	26 wks	Insulin detemir and insulin aspart	0.9 (5/537)
			Biphasic insulin aspart	0/178
Rosenstock, 2008[40]	RCT	52 wks	Insulin detemir	1.7 (5/291)
			Insulin glargine	2.7 (8/291)
Meneghini (PREDICTIVE) 2007[176]	RCT	26 wks	Insulin detemir - Algorithm care	0.26 events per patient years
			Insulin detemir - Standard care	0.20 events per patient years
Haak, 2005[33]	RCT	26 wks	Insulin detemir	<2% in both arms (numbers NR)
			NPH insulin	
Marre (PREDICTIVE) 2009[18]	Prospective cohort	52 wks	Insulin detemir	0.3 (4/1129)
G. Insulin glargine studies: long-acting				
Buse, 2011[36]	RCT	2.5 yrs follow-up	Insulin glargine (long-acting)	2.9 (12/419)
			Insulin lispro 75/25 mix	4.2 (20/473)
Rosenstock, 2009[35]	RCT	5 yrs	Insulin glargine (long-acting)	7.6 (38/513)
			NPH insulin (intermediate acting)	11.1 (55/504)
Russell-Jones, 2009[54]	RCT	26 wks	Insulin glargine (long-acting) added to metformin and sulfonylurea)	0/232
			Liraglutide added to metformin and sulfonylurea)	2.2 (5/230)
			Placebo added to metformin and sulfonylurea)	0/114

Study and year	Study type	Study duration	Intervention(s) Control	Hypoglycemia Incidence % (n/N)
Rosenstock, 2008[40]	RCT	52 wks	Insulin glargine	2.7 (8/291)
			Insulin detemir	1.7 (5/291)
Kennedy, 2006[37]	RCT	24 wks	Insulin glargine, usual and active titration	3 (228/7607)
			Insulin glargine, usual titration	0.09 events per patient-year
			Insulin glargine, active titration	0.14 events per patient-year
Standl, 2006[180]	RCT	24 wks	Insulin glargine, morning administration + Glimepiride (G) 2-4 mg	1.3 (4/299)
			Insulin glargine, bedtime administration + G 2-4 mg	0.7 (2/281)
Davies, 2005[38]	RCT	24 wks	Insulin glargine algorithm 1 (investigator led)	0.9 (21/2315)
			Insulin glargine algorithm 2 (performed by study subjects)	1.1 (25/2273)
Heine, 2005[42]	RCT	26 wks	Adjunct Insulin glargine (long-acting) added to oral therapy (metformin and sulfonylurea	1.5 (4/267)
			Adjunct Exenatide added to oral therapy (metformin and sulfonylurea)	1.4 (4/282)
Fritsche, 2003[44]	RCT	24 wks	Bedtime Insulin glargine + G	1.8 (4/227)
			Morning Insulin glargine + G	2.1 (5/236)
			NPH insulin (intermediate acting) +G	2.6 (6/232)
Riddle, 2003[41]	RCT	24 wks	Insulin glargine (long-acting)	2.5 (9/367)
			NPH insulin (intermediate acting)	1.8 (7/389)
Rosenstock, 2001[39]	RCT	28 wks	Insulin glargine (long-acting)	0.4 (1/259)
			NPH insulin (intermediate acting)	2.3 (6/259)
H. Non-specific Insulin studies				
UK Hypoglycemia Group 2007[190]	Prospective cohort	9-12 mos	Treated with insulin for <2 years	~7.0* (6/89)
			Treated with insulin for >5 years	~25.0* (19/77)
			Sulfonylurea	7.0 (8/108)
Murata, 2005[19]	Prospective cohort	41 wks	Long-acting insulin	5.5 (19/344)
Nichols, 2010[26]	Retrospective cohort	49 mos	All types (regular, quick-acting, NPH, mixed, etc.) Hypoglycemia requiring a medical contact occurred in 1.9% of patients in the first year of insulin use, but by the fifth year the rate had fallen to 0,4%. No cases of required hospitalization.	
Asche, 2008[23]	Retrospective cohort	395 days of followup	Insulin with sulfonylurea	2.8 (3/106)
			Insulin with thiazolidinedione	4.3 (8/187)
			Sulfonylurea monotherapy	2.6 (55/2117)
			Thiazolidinedione monotherapy	1.7 (12/702)
			Metformin	0/2326
Leese, 2003[25]	Retrospective cohort	NR	Insulin	7.3 (66/901) 11.8/100 patient yrs [95% CI 9.5 to 14.1]

*extracted from graph

Table 3c. Sulfonylurea Studies

Study and year	Study type	Study duration	Intervention (daily dose) Control	Hypoglycemia Incidence % (n/N)
Arechavaleta, 2011[52]	RCT	30 wks	Adjunct Glimepiride 1-6 mg added to metformin	1.5 (8/519)
			Adjunct Sitagliptin 100 mg added to metformin	0.2 (1/516)
Garber, 2011[51]	RCT	52 wks	Glimepiride 8 mg	0/248
			Liragultide 1.2 mg	0/251
			Liragultide 1.8 mg	0/247
Matthews, 2010[49]	RCT	2 yrs	Adjunct Glimepiride 2-6 mg added to metformin	1.8 (15/1546)
			Adjunct Vildagliptin 100 mg added to metformin	0/1553
Seck, 2010;[50] Nauck, 2007[177]	RCT	2 yrs	Adjunct Glipizde 5 mg added to metformin	Non-med. Assist. 1.5 (9/584) Med. Assist. 1.5 (9/584)
			Adjunct Sitagliptin 100 mg added to metformin	Non-med. Assist. 0.2 (1/588) Med. Assist. 0.2 (1/588)
Marre, 2009[175]	RCT	52 wks	Glimepiride 2-4 mg + liragultide 0.6 mg	0/233
			Glimepiride 2-4 mg + liragultide 1.2 mg	0/228
			Glimepiride 2-4 mg + liragultide 1.8 mg	1.7 (4/234)
			Glimepiride 2-4 mg	0/114
			Rosiglitazone 8 mg + Glimepiride 2-4 mg	0/232
Nauck, 2009[53] LEAD-2	RCT	26 wks	Glimepiride 4 mg plus Metformin	0/242
			Liragultide 0.6 mg plus Metformin	0/242
			Liragultide 1.2 mg plus Metformin	0/241
			Liragultide 1.8 mg plus Metformin	0/242
			Placebo plus Metformin	0/121
Russell-Jones, 2009[54] LEAD-5	RCT	26 wks	Insulin glargine (long-acting) added to metformin and sulfonylurea)	0/232
			Liraglutide added to metformin and sulfonylurea)	2.2 (5/230)
			Placebo added to metformin and sulfonylurea)	0/114
Chou, 2008[55]	RCT	28 wks	Glimepiride (G) 1–4 mg	0/225
			Rosiglitazone (R) 4-8 mg	0/232
			R to 4 mg + G to 4 mg (Regimen A)	0.4 (1/225)
			R to 8 mg + G to 4 mg (Regimen B)	0.9 (2/219)
Standl, 2006[180]	RCT	24 wks	Glimepiride 2-4 mg + Insulin glargine, morning administration +	.3 (4/299)
			Glimepiride 2-4 mg + Insulin glargine, bedtime administration	0.7 (2/281)
Heine, 2005[42]	RCT	26 wks	Adjunct Exenatide 20 µg added to oral therapy (metformin and sulfonylurea)	1.4 (4/282)
			Adjunct Insulin glargine added to oral therapy (metformin and sulfonylurea)	1.5 (4/267)

Study and year	Study type	Study duration	Intervention (daily dose) Control	Hypoglycemia Incidence % (n/N)
Kendall, 2005[56]	RCT	30 wks	Adjunct Exenatide 20 µg to oral therapy (metformin and sulfonylurea)	0/241
			Adjunct Exenatide 10 µg to oral therapy (metformin and sulfonylurea)	0.4 (1/245)
			Adjunct Placebo to oral therapy (metformin and sulfonylurea)	0/247
Drouin, 2004[32]	RCT	10 mos	Gliclazide modified release 30–120 mg	0/401
			Gliclazide 80–120 mg	0.3 (1/399)
Schernthaner, 2004[57]	RCT	27 wks	Glimepiride 1–6 mg	0/440
			Gliclazide 30–120 mg	0/405
Fritsche, 2003[44]	RCT	24 wks	Glimepiride 3 mg + NPH insulin	2.6 (6/232)
			Glimepiride 3 mg + Bedtime Insulin glargine	1.8 (4/227)
			Glimepiride 3 mg + Morning Insulin glargine	2.1 (5/236)
UK Hypoglycemia Group[190]	Prospective cohort	9-12 mos	Sulfonylurea	7.0 (8/108)
			Treated with insulin for <2 years	~7.0* (6/89)
			Treated with insulin for >5 years	~25.0* (19/77)
Holstein, 2001[17]	Prospective population-based cohort	4 yrs	Overall	5.6/100,000 inhabitants/yr
			Glimepiride 2 mg	0.3 (6/1768) 0.86/1000 person yrs
			Gilbenclamide 7 mg	2.2 (38/1721) 5.6/1000 person yrs
Asche, 2008[23]	Retrospective cohort	395 days of followup	Sulfonylurea monotherapy	2.6 (55/2117)
			Sulfonylurea with Insulin	2.8 (3/106)
			Thiazolidinedione with insulin	4.3 (8/187)
			Thiazolidinedione monotherapy	1.7 (12/702)
			Metformin	0/2326
Bodmer, 2008[24] N=50,048 of which 73 had severe hypoglycemia	Retrospective cohort with nested case control	NR/NA	Sulfonylurea	110/100,000 person yrs (22 patients on monotherapy [16 gliclazide, 5 glibenclamide, 1 glimepiride], 11 combined with metformin)
Leese, 2003[25]	Retrospective cohort	NR/NA	Sulfonylurea	0.8 (23/2823) 0.09/100 patient yrs [95%CI 0.6 to 1.3]
Stahl, 1999[28]	Retrospective case series	12 yrs	Long-acting Sulfonylureas	2.7 (16/594) (15 glibenclamide, 1 chlorpropamide)
			Short-acting Sulfonylureas	0.9 (12/1334)
			Glibornuride	*0.9 (10/1138)*
			Gliclazide	*1.0 (2/196)*
			Any Sulfonylurea	1.5 (28/1928)

* Not reported, estimated from figure

Table 3d. Metformin (Biguanides) Studies

Study and year	Study type	Study duration	Intervention (daily dose) Control	Hypoglycemia Incidence % (n/N)
Arechavaleta, 2011[52]	RCT	30 wks	Metformin with adjunct glimepiride 1-6 mg	1.5 (8/519)
			Metformin with adjunct sitagliptin 100 mg	0.2 (1/516)
Matthews, 2010[49]	RCT	2 yrs	Metformin with adjunct glimepiride 2-6 mg	1.8 (15/1546)
			Metformin with adjunct vildagliptin 100 mg	0/1553
Olansky, 2011[178]	RCT	44 wks	Metformin up to 2000 mg	0/625
			Metformin and sitagliptin up to 100 mg	0/621
Aschner, 2010[60]	RCT	24 wks	Metformin 2000 mg	0/522
			Sitagliptin 100 mg	0.4 (2/528)
Pratley, 2010[179]	RCT	26 wks	Metformin with adjunct sitagliptin 100 mg	0/219
			Metformin with adjunct liragultide 1.2 mg	0.4 (1/225)
			Metformin with adjunct liragultide 1.8 mg	0/221
Seck, 2010;[50] Nauck, 2007[177]	RCT	2 yrs	Metformin with adjunct Sitagliptin 100 mg	Non-med. Assist. 0.2 (1/588) Med. Assist. 0.2 (1/588)
			Metformin with adjunct Glipizde 5 mg	Non-med. Assist. 1.5 (9/584) Med. Assist. 1.5 (9/584)
Nauck, 2009[53] LEAD-2	RCT	26 wks	Liragultide 0.6 mg plus Metformin	0/242
			Liragultide 1.2 mg plus Metformin	0/241
			Liragultide 1.8 mg plus Metformin	0/242
			Glimepiride 4 mg plus Metformin	0/242
			Placebo plus Metformin	0/121
Raskin, 2009[31]	RCT	26 wks	Metformin 2000 mg and repaglinide bid (maximum dose 4 mg)	0/177
			Metformin tid (doses 1000,500,1000 mg) and repaglinide tid (maximum doses 4,2, and 4 mg)	0/178
			Metformin 2000 mg and rosiglitazone bid (maximum dose 4 mg)	0/206
Russell-Jones, 2009[54] LEAD-5	RCT	26 wks	Insulin glargine (long-acting) added to metformin and sulfonylurea)	0/232
			Liraglutide added to metformin and sulfonylurea)	2.2 (5/230)
			Placebo added to metformin and sulfonylurea)	0/114
Williams-Herman, 2009;[113] Goldstein, 2007[181] *Patients could be on oral meds*	RCT	54 wks	Metformin (M) 500 mg	1.1 (2/182)
			Metformin 1000 mg	0/182
			Sitagliptin 100 mg	0/179
			Sitagliptin 50 mg + Metformin 500 mg	0/190
			Placebo/ Metformin 1000 mg	0/176
Zinman, 2009	RCT	26 wks	Metformin (M) 2 g + rosiglitazone (R) 8 mg and liraglutide 1.2 mg	0/178
			M+R and liraglutide 1.8 mg	0/178
			M+R and placebo	0/177

Study and year	Study type	Study duration	Intervention (daily dose) Control	Hypoglycemia Incidence % (n/N)
Bolli, 2008[172]	RCT	24 wks	Adjunct Pioglitazone 30 mg + metformin ≥ 1500 mg	0/281
			Adjunct Vildagliptin 100 mg + metformin ≥ 1500 mg	0/295
Heine, 2005[42]	RCT	26 wks	Adjunct Exenatide 20 µg added to oral therapy (metformin and sulfonylurea)	1.4 (4/282)
			Adjunct Insulin glargine added to oral therapy (metformin and sulfonylurea)	1.5 (4/267)
Kendall, 2005[56]	RCT	30 wks	Adjunct Exenatide 20 µg to oral therapy (metformin and sulfonylurea)	0/241
			Adjunct Exenatide 10 µg to oral therapy (metformin and sulfonylurea)	0.4 (1/245)
			Adjunct Placebo to oral therapy (metformin and sulfonylurea)	0/247
UKPDS 28 1998[191]	RCT	3 yrs	Adjunct metformin to 2250 mg + sulfonylurea	0.3 (1/291)
			Sulfonylurea	0/300
Bodmer, 2008[24] N=50,048 of which 73 had severe hypoglycemia	Retrospective cohort with nested case-control	NR/NA	Metformin	60/100,000 person yrs (3 patients on monotherapy, 11 combined with sulfonylurea)
Asche, 2008[23]	Retrospective cohort	395 days of followup	Metformin	0/2326
			Sulfonylurea monotherapy	2.6 (55/2117)
			Sulfonylurea with Insulin	2.8 (3/106)
			Thiazolidinedione monotherapy	1.7 (12/702)
			Thiazolidinedione with insulin	4.3 (8/187)
Leese, 2003[25]	Retrospective cohort	NR/NA	Metformin or diet	0.05/100 patient yrs [95% CI 0.01 to 0.2]

Table 3e. Dipeptidyl-Peptidase-4 Inhibitors (DPP-4) Studies

Study and year	Study type	Study duration	Intervention (daily dose) Control	Hypoglycemia Incidence % (n/N)
Arechavaleta, 2011[52]	RCT	30 wks	Adjunct Sitagliptin 100 mg added to metformin	0.2 (1/516)
			Adjunct Glimepiride 1-6 mg added to metformin	1.5 (8/519)
Matthews, 2010[49]	RCT	2 yrs	Adjunct Vildagliptin 100 mg added to metformin	0/1553
			Adjunct Glimepiride 2-6 mg added to metformin	1.8 (15/1546)
Olansky, 2011[178]	RCT	44 wks	Sitagliptin up to 100 mg and metformin up to 2000 mg	0/625
			Metformin up to 2000 mg	0/621
Aschner, 2010[60]	RCT	24 wks	Sitagliptin 100 mg	0.4 (2/528)
			Metformin 2000 mg	0/522

Study and year	Study type	Study duration	Intervention (daily dose) Control	Hypoglycemia Incidence % (n/N)
Pratley, 2010[179]	RCT	26 wks	Adjunct Sitagliptin 100 mg added to metformin	0/219
			Adjunct Liragultide 1.2 mg added to metformin	0.4 (1/225)
			Adjunct Liragultide 1.8 mg added to metformin	0/221
Seck 2010;[50] Nauck, 2007[177]	RCT	2 yrs	Adjunct Sitagliptin 100 mg added to metformin	Non-med. Assist. 0.2 (1/588) Med. Assist. 0.2 (1/588)
			Adjunct Glipizde 5 mg added to metformin	Non-med. Assist. 1.5 (9/584) Med. Assist. 1.5 (9/584)
Williams-Herman, 2009;[113] Goldstein, 2007[181] *Patients could be on oral meds*	RCT	54 wks	Sitagliptin 100 mg	0/179
			Sitagliptin 50 mg + Metformin 500 mg	0/190
			Sitagliptin 50 mg + Metformin 1000 mg	0/182
			Metformin 500 mg	1.1 (2/182)
			Metformin 1000 mg	0/182
			Placebo/ Metformin 1000 mg	0/176
Bolli 2008/2009[172, 173]	RCT	24 wks	Adjunct Vildagliptin 100 mg + metformin ≥ 1500 mg	0/295
			Adjunct Pioglitazone 30 mg + metformin ≥ 1500 mg	0/281
Aschner, 2006[136] *Patients could be on oral meds*	RCT	24 wks	Sitagliptin 100 mg	0/238
			Sitagliptin 200 mg	0/250
			Placebo	0/253

Table 3f. Glucagon-like Peptide-1 (GLP-1) Analogs Studies

Study and year	Study type	Study duration	Intervention (daily dose) Control	Hypoglycemia Incidence % (n/N)
Garber, 2011[51]	RCT	52 wks	Liragultide 1.2 mg	0/251
			Liragultide 1.8 mg	0/247
			Glimepiride 8 mg	0/248
Pratley, 2010[179]	RCT	26 wks	Adjunct Liragultide 1.2 mg added to metformin	0.4 (1/225)
			Adjunct Liragultide 1.8 mg added to metformin	0/221
			Adjunct Sitagliptin 100 mg added to metformin	0/219
Marre, 2009[175]	RCT	52 wks	Liragultide 0.6 mg + glimepiride 2-4 mg	0/233
			Liragultide 1.2 mg + glimepiride 2-4 mg	0/228
			Liragultide 1.8 mg + glimepiride 2-4 mg	1.7 (4/234)
			Glimepiride 2-4 mg	0/114
			Rosiglitazone 8 mg + Glimepiride 2-4 mg	0/232
Nauck, 2009[53] LEAD-2	RCT	26 wks	Liragultide 0.6 mg plus Metformin	0/242
			Liragultide 1.2 mg plus Metformin	0/241
			Liragultide 1.8 mg plus Metformin	0/242
			Glimepiride 4 mg plus Metformin	0/242
			Placebo plus Metformin	0/121

Study and year	Study type	Study duration	Intervention (daily dose) Control	Hypoglycemia Incidence % (n/N)
Russell-Jones, 2009[54] LEAD-5	RCT	26 wks	Liraglutide added to metformin and sulfonylurea)	2.2 (5/230)
			Insulin glargine (long-acting) added to metformin and sulfonylurea)	0/232
			Placebo added to metformin and sulfonylurea)	0/114
Zinman, 2009[182]	RCT	26 wks	Liragultide 1.2 mg plus Metformin (M) 2 g + rosiglitazone (R) 8 mg	0/178
			Liragultide 1.8 mg and M + R	0/178
			Placebo and M + R	0/177
Heine, 2005[42]	RCT	26 wks	Adjunct Exenatide 20 µg added to oral therapy (metformin and sulfonylurea)	1.4 (4/282)
			Adjunct Insulin glargine added to oral therapy (metformin and sulfonylurea)	1.5 (4/267)
Kendall, 2005[56]	RCT	30 wks	Adjunct Exenatide 20 µg to oral therapy (metformin and sulfonylurea)	0/241
			Adjunct Exenatide 10 µg to oral therapy (metformin and sulfonylurea)	0.4 (1/245)
			Adjunct Placebo to oral therapy (metformin and sulfonylurea)	0/247

* One event in the liraglutide1.8 mg group occurred after regular insulin was infused during the extension period (post 52 weeks)

Table 3g. Bari 2D, Insulin Sensitization versus Insulin Provision

Study and year	Study type	Study duration	Intervention Control	Hypoglycemia Incidence % (n/N)
BARI 2D*[58]	RCT	5.3 yrs	Insulin sensitization therapy	5.9 (68/1153)
			Insulin-provision therapy	9.2 (106/1154) P=0.003

* Medication use among all patients was as follows: metformin 54%; sulfonylurea 53%; insulin 28%; any thiazolidinedione 19%; rosiglitazone 10%.

Table 3h. Amylin Analog Studies

Study and year	Study type	Study duration	Intervention Control	Hypoglycemia Incidence % (n/N)
Ratner, 2002[34]	RCT	52 wks	Adjunct Pramlintide 30 µg tid to insulin therapy (some patients were also on oral agents)	1.6 (2/122)
			Adjunct Pramlintide 75 µg tid to insulin therapy (some patients were also on oral agents)	0.7 (1/136)
			Adjunct Pramlintide 150 µg tid to insulin therapy (some patients were also on oral agents)	1.4 (2/144)
			Adjunct Placebo to insulin therapy (some patients were also on oral agents)	1.5 (2/136)

Study and year	Study type	Study duration	Intervention Control	Hypoglycemia Incidence % (n/N)
Pencek, 2010[20]	Prospective cohort	6 mos	Adjunct Pramlintide to insulin therapy (some patients were also on oral agents)	<u>Patient-ascertained severe hypoglycemia</u> 1) adjustment period (0–3 months) 2.8% (n=531); 2) maintenance period (>3–6 months) 0.4% (n=387) <u>Medically-assisted severe hypoglycemia</u> 1) adjustment period (0–3 months) 0.4% (n=531); 2) maintenance period (>3–6 months) 0.3% (n=387)

Table 3i. Glinide Studies

Study and year	Study type	Study duration	Intervention Control	Hypoglycemia Incidence* % (n/N)
Raskin, 2009[31]	RCT	26 wks	Repaglinide bid (maximum dose 4 mg) / metformin 2000 mg	0/177
			Repaglinide tid (maximum doses 4,2, and 4 mg)/metformin tid (doses of 1000,500,1000 mg)	0/178
			Rosiglitazone bid (maximum doses 4 mg)/ metformin 2000 mg	0/206
Saloranta, 2002[59] Serious events rare (Not reported) *Diet alone subjects*	RCT	24 wks	Nateglinide 30 mg tid	0/166
			Nateglinide 60 mg tid	0/175
			Nateglinide 1200 mg tid	0/171
			Placebo tid	0/163

* Requiring assistance from an outside party

Table 3j. Thiazolidinedione Studies

Study and year	Study type	Study duration	Intervention (daily dose) Control	Hypoglycemia Incidence % (n/N)
Marre, 2009[175]	RCT	26 wks	Rosiglitazone 8 mg + Glimepiride 2-4 mg	0/232
			Glimepiride 2-4 mg + liragultide 0.6 mg	0/233
			Glimepiride 2-4 mg + liragultide 1.2 mg	0/228
			Glimepiride 2-4 mg + liragultide 1.8 mg	1.7 (4/234)
			Glimepiride 2-4 mg	0/114

Study and year	Study type	Study duration	Intervention (daily dose) Control	Hypoglycemia Incidence % (n/N)
Raskin, 2009[31]	RCT	26 wks	Rosiglitazone bid (maximum dose 4 mg) / metformin 2000 mg	0/206
			Repaglinide bid (maximum dose 4 mg) / metformin 2000 mg	0/177
			Repaglinide tid (maximum doses 4,2, and 4 mg)/metformin tid (doses 1000-500-1000 mg)	0/178
Zinman, 2009[182]	RCT	26 wks	Rosiglitazone (R) 8 mg + Metformin (M) 2 g and liraglutide 1.2 mg	0/178
			R + M and liraglutide 1.8 mg	0/178
			R + M and placebo	0/177
Bolli, 2008[172]	RCT	24 wks	Adjunct Pioglitazone 30 mg + metformin ≥ 1500 mg	0/281
			Adjunct Vildagliptin 100 mg + metformin ≥ 1500 mg	0/295
Chou, 2008[55] *Drug-naive subjects*	RCT	28 wks	Glimepiride (G) 1–4 mg	0/232
			Rosiglitazone (R) 4-8 mg	0/225
			R to 4 mg + G to 4 mg (Regimen A)	0.4 (1/225)
			R to 8 mg + G to 4 mg (Regimen B)	0.9 (2/219)
Dormandy, 2005[174] (PROactive)	RCT	34.5 mos	Adjunct Pioglitazone 15-45 mg + other glucose lowering drugs	0.73 (19/2605)
			Adjunct Placebo + other glucose lowering drugs	0.42 (11/2633)
Asche, 2008[23]	Retrospective cohort	395 days of followup	Thiazolidinedione monotherapy	1.7 (12/702)
			Thiazolidinedione with insulin	4.3 (8/187)
			Sulfonylurea monotherapy	2.6 (55/2117)
			Sulfonylurea with Insulin	2.8 (3/106)
			Metformin	0

Table 3k. Studies in Which Patients are on a Variety of Medications

Study and year	Study type	Study duration	Intervention Control	Hypoglycemia Incidence % (n/N)
Davis, 2010[16]	Prospective community-based cohort	6.4 yrs	Several, not described	8.4 (52/616) 1.7 per 100 patient-years
Quilliam, 2011[183]	Retrospective cohort of working-age patients	Patients who were represented for at least one year in a database	The most common classes of OHAs were metformin (75.7%), sulfonylureas (42.3%), and thiazolidinediones (33.3%). Insulin use in addition to OHA use was relatively infrequent, (6.0%)	3.5 (653/18,657) 1.5 per 100 patient-years

Table 3l. Management (Self vs. GP or Nurse Management) Studies

Study and year	Study type	Study duration	Intervention Control	Hypoglycemia Incidence % (n/N)
Barnett, 2008[171]	RCT	27 wks	Gliclazide - self-monitoring of blood glucose (SMBG)	0/311
			Gliclazide – Non-SMBG	0/299
Meneghini (PREDICTIVE) 2007[176]	RCT	26 wks	Insulin detemir - Algorithm care	0.26 events per patient years
			Insulin detemir - Standard care	0.20 events per patient years

Table 4. Risk Factor Data Table for Key Question #2

Study Location Funding Age/Sex	Study Design Analysis Definition of Severe # of Patients	Risk Factors for Severe Hypoglycemia OR Patient Characteristics If No Formal Risk Factor Analysis			
		Univariate analysis (RAE – risk of any event, RRE – risk of repeated events)			
			RAE OR 95% CI	p value	RRE RR 95% CI	p value
Akram, 2006[64]	Cross-sectional survey				
Denmark	Multivariate	Age	1.01 0.99–1.04	0.366	0.98 0.97–1.00	0.030
		Diabetes duration	1.02 0.98–1.06	0.400	0.96 0.94–0.98	< 0.001
Danish Research Medical Council	The need for assistance from another person to treat the condition in the preceding year	Diabetes duration prior to insulin start	0.98 0.93–1.02	0.403	0.93 0.91–0.96	< 0.001
		Duration of insulin therapy	1.07 1.01–1.13	0.018	0.99 0.96–1.02	0.370
		Impaired awareness	2.66 1.55–4.56	< 0.001	1.18 0.87–1.59	0.229
66/men and women	401 surveys completed, 66 at least one event, 178 total episodes, overall incidence of severe hypoglycemia 0.44 episodes/ person year	Insulin regimens:				
		Twice daily	2.89 0.67–12.6	0.157	0.45 0.25–0.87	0.017
		Three times daily	2.07 0.27–16.1	0.489	0.18 0.04–0.82	0.027
		Four times daily	4.81 1.05–22.1	0.043	0.54 0.28–1.03	0.059
		Retinopathy (untreated)	0.99 0.56–1.78	0.979	0.63 0.45–0.86	0.004
		Peripheral neuropathy (asymptomatic)	1.64 0.80–3.39	0.181	2.00 1.33–2.99	0.001
		Peripheral neuropathy (symptomatic)	1.69 0.92–3.11	0.089	1.42 0.97–2.07	0.071
		Hypertension	0.57 0.33–0.97	0.039	1.40 1.03–1.90	0.033
		Hypertension therapy:				
		RAS blocking	0.89 0.31–2.54	0.826	0.65 0.39–1.08	0.096
		Non-RAS blocking drugs	1.55 0.65–3.71	0.323	0.38 0.24–0.59	< 0.001
		Combination of both	0.63 0.27–1.43	0.266	0.65 0.44–0.95	0.027
		Macrovascular complication (stroke, MI)	1.14 0.57–2.27	0.719	1.78 1.28–2.48	0.001
		Metformin	0.51 0.25–1.01	0.052	1.05 0.72–1.55	0.789
		Marital status (married)	2.57 1.32–5.01	0.006	1.19 0.80–1.79	0.393
		Exercise (strenuous)	0.49 0.19–1.31	0.154	2.06 1.33–3.18	0.001
		Smoking	0.74 0.38–1.46	0.389	1.43 1.02–2.02	0.041
		Use of tranquilizers	1.66 0.93–2.98	0.087	1.57 1.17–2.12	0.003
		Multivariate analysis - *Risk of any event*				
		Impaired awareness 3 fold increased risk of any event				
		Long duration of DM (per 10 years) 2 fold increased risk of any event				
		Being married 2 fold increased risk of any event				
		Rate of severe hypoglycemia (risk of repeated events)				
		Peripheral neuropathy 3x increased rate				
		Long duration of DM (per 10 years) prior to insulin therapy 3x decreased rate				
		Tx with RAS blocking drugs ½ rate of severe hypoglycemia				

Study Location Funding Age/Sex	Study Design Analysis Definition of Severe # of Patients	Risk Factors for Severe Hypoglycemia OR Patient Characteristics If No Formal Risk Factor Analysis		
Alvarez Guisasola, 2008[85] Multicenter (7 countries) Industry 63/men and women	Observational, cross-sectional, multicentre study Unadjusted Based on answer to question "Have you ever felt symptoms of hypoglycemia (low blood sugar) in the past year? (iii) felt you needed assistance of others to manage symptoms (iv) needed medical attention, ambulance, ER, saw doctor or nurse	**Patient reported outcomes and HbA1c goal status**		
		Characteristic	patients at goal	patients not at goal	p value
		Hypoglycemic symptoms who felt the need for assistance, including medical attention, to manage symptoms	5.8 (11/190)	4.8 (22/462)	0.0152*
		*This p value was combined with other hypoglycemia symptom severities		
Asplund, 1991[105] Sweden NR 75/men and women	Case-control 2 – matched on gender and age Median BG 1.7 mmol/l 11 patients comatose, 3 reduced consciousness, five fully alert but with signs/symptoms of hypoglycemia and sought medical attention 422 patients on glipizide, - 19 with severe hypoglycemia 844 controls		Cases	Controls	P value
		Duration of diabetes (months)	36 (14-48)	75 (52-108)	0.004
		Duration of sulfonylurea treatment (months)	14 (6-43)	51 (34-75)	0.004
		Duration of glipizide treatment (months)	12 (3-26)	41.5 (26-59)	<0.001
		Glipizide dose (mg day)	10 (5-15)	10 (5-15)	NS
		Number of concomitant drugs (excluding glipizide)	5 (3.5-5)	2 (1-1)	<0.001
		Cardiac Disorders, Renal Disorders, Liver Disorders, Cerebral Disorders all more common in hypoglycemia group Only significant in renal disease: OR 4.0 95% CI 1.2-13.1 Circulatory disease 14/19 (74%) Hepatic failure (moderate) 2/19 (11%) Other meds taken by cases: Diuretic 13/19 (68%); Cardiac clycosides 6/19; Benzodiazepines 5/19; NSAIDS 4/19; beta-blocker 4/19; salicylates 4/19 Significant drug ORs (cases vs. controls): Any diuretic OR=8.5 (CI 1.7-29.3) Benzodiazepines OR=10.0 (CI 1.4-71.8)		

Predictors and Consequences of Severe Hypoglycemia in Adults with Diabetes – Systematic Review of the Evidence

Study Location Funding Age/Sex	Study Design Analysis Definition of Severe # of Patients	Risk Factors for Severe Hypoglycemia OR Patient Characteristics If No Formal Risk Factor Analysis
Bodmer, 2008[24] UK based General practice Research Database UK Industry 61/men and women	Nested case control within retrospective cohort Unadjusted for severe hypoglycemia, adjusted for generic hypoglycemia Hypoglycemia leading to an emergency hospitalization or death 2,025 case subjects, 7,278 matched controls 73 out of 2,025 had severe hypoglycemia	"Numbers too small for a meaningful model." – formal risk analysis not performed Of 73 case subjects 35 were on insulin (26 were on insulin only and 9 used insulin in combination with an oral antidiabetes drug) 22 used sulfonylureas only 3 metformin only 11 a combination of sulfonylureas and metformin 2 were past users of antidiabetes drugs. Among 22 users of sulfonlyureas only, 16 used gliclazide, 5 glibenclamide, and 1 glimepiride, and 17 used a high dose and 5 a low dose.

Bruce, 2009[92]
 	
Fremantle (older patients with cognitive impairment/ dementia)
 	
Australia
 	
Government (Initial Fremantle) and Government/ Industry (this study)
 	
76/men and women
	Prospective Cohort
	
	Univariate and multivariate
	
	Cox proportional hazards; Negative binomial regression model
	
	Severe hypoglycemia
	Answer yes to "Have you ever had to go the hospital because of a hypoglycemic attack?" or "Have you ever had a serious hypoglycemic attack that made you go unconscious?"
	Health service use for hypoglycemia (HSH)(used as severe hypoglycemia during followup)
	An event requiring ambulance and/or emergency department attendance and/or hospitalization for hypoglycemia as the primary diagnosis
	
	302, 27 had HSH during followup
		At study entry:
		No significant independent associations between dementia and any measure of hypoglycemia, however:
		Cognitive impairment without dementia:
		  Self reported severe hypoglycemia (OR 2.96 (1.05-8.33))
		  Doctor verified neuroglycopenia (OR 5.10 (1.46-17.87))
		  HSH (OR 9.65 (1.65-56.60))
		
		Significant Risk Factors
		Time to first HSH
		
		          HR 95% CI p value
		Dementia 3.02 (1.07-8.53) 0.037
		Insulin therapy 2.77 (1.18-6.46) 0.019
		Low BMI 5.94 (1.85-19.06) 0.003
		Inability to self manage medications 4.19 (1.43-12.25) 0.009
		History of self reported severe hypoglycemia 3.51 (1.15-10.76) 0.028
		
		Frequency of HSH
		
		          RR 95% CI p value
		Dementia 20.26 (6.00-68.44) <0.001
		Insulin therapy 14.60 (3.49-61.12) <0.001
		Renal Impairment 4.70 (1.02-21.70) 0.048

Predictors and Consequences of Severe Hypoglycemia in Adults with Diabetes – Systematic Review of the Evidence

Study Location Funding Age/Sex	Study Design Analysis Definition of Severe # of Patients	Risk Factors for Severe Hypoglycemia OR Patient Characteristics If No Formal Risk Factor Analysis	HR (95% CI)	p value
Davis, 2010[16]	Prospective cohort Univariate and multivariate	**Univariate associates**	**HR (95% CI)**	**p value**
		Age 65 yr or older	1.15 (0.65-2.02)	0.63
Fremantle		Male sex	0.97 (0.56-1.67)	0.90
(everyone)	An episode in which a patient with	BMI <29.0 kg/m^2	0.97 (0.56-1.68)	0.92
	a subnormal blood/plasma/serum	Education attainment higher than primary level	1.65 (0.78-3.51)	0.19
Australia	glucose required health service use	English ability (not fluent)	0.53 (0.19-1.48)	0.23
	and hypoglycemia was the primary	Any exercise in past 2 wks	0.60 (0.34-1.04)	0.07
Government	diagnosis	Daily alcohol consumption of three or more standard drinks	1.38 (0.55-3.46)	0.50
(Initial		GAD ab positive	4.41 (1.75-11.10)	0.002
Fremantle) and	616	Diabetes duration > or equal to 8 yr	2.92 (1.60-5.32)	<0.001
Industry (this	52 had 66 episodes of severe	FSG >or equal to 8.0 mmol/liter	1.32 (0.73-2.38)	0.35
study)	hypoglycemia	AbA1c > or equal to 7.0%	2.11 (1.13-3.95)	0.020
		Sulfonylurea treatment (vs. lifestyle/other oral agents)	2.50 (1.16-5.38)	0.019
67/men and		Insulin treatment (+/- oral agents)	4.29 (2.44-7.55)	<0.001
women		Time on insulin (increase of 1 yr)	1.42 (1.24-1.63)	<0.001
		Blood glucose self monitoring	1.01 (0.48-2.15)	0.98
		History of severe hypoglycemia	6.59 (2.62-16.60)	<0.001
		eGFR <60 ml.min per 1.73 m^2	2.90 (1.68-5.00)	<0.001
		Peripheral neuropathy	2.89 (1.60-5.21)	<0.001
		Orthostatic hypotension	1.74 (0.99-1.15)	0.34
		QTc interval (increase of 10 msec^0.5)	1.05 (0.95-1.15)	0.34
		Five or more prescribed medications	1.84 (1.07-3.17)	0.028
		Anticoagulant therapy	2.93 (1.06-8.13)	0.039
		Regular aspirin use (> or equal to 75 mg/d)	1.31 (0.74-2.31)	0.36
		NSAID treatment	1.29 (0.61-2.74)	0.51
		Allopurinol treatment	1.62 (0.65-4.08)	0.30
		Fibrate treatment	1.86 (0.74-4.67)	0.19
		Beta-blocker treatment	1.26 (0.63-2.51)	0.51
		Hospitalized in 1998	1.77 (1.03-3.05)	0.039
		Independent associates	**HR (95% CI)**	**p value**
		Time on insulin (increase of 1 yr)	1.33 (1.15-1.53)	<0.001
		History of severe hypoglycemia	5.66 (2.21-14.50)	<0.001
		eGFR <60 ml/min per 1.73 m^2	2.39 (1.37-4.15)	0.002
		Peripheral neuropathy	2.44 (1.33-4.47)	0.004
		Education attainment higher than primary level	2.34 (1.09-5.04)	0.029

Predictors and Consequences of Severe Hypoglycemia in Adults with Diabetes – Systematic Review of the Evidence

Study Location Funding Age/Sex	Study Design Analysis Definition of Severe # of Patients	Risk Factors for Severe Hypoglycemia OR Patient Characteristics If No Formal Risk Factor Analysis		
Davis, 2011[93]	Followup of Fremantle Prospective cohort patients	Independent baseline predictors of time to first severe hypoglycemic event and frequency of severe hypoglycemia during follow-up		
		Time to first event	**Hazard ratio (95% CI)**	**p value**
Patients taken from Fremantle	Multivariate	Time on insulin (increase of 1 yr)	1.33 (1.15–1.53)	0.001
		History of severe hypoglycemia	5.48 (2.05–14.64)	0.001
Australia	Requiring documented health service use	eGFR _ 60 ml/min per 1.73m2	2.63 (1.46–4.73)	0.001
		Peripheral neuropathy	2.57 (1.36–4.84)	0.004
Government (Initial Fremantle) and Industry (this study)	602 patients ACE genotyped, 49 patients reported 63 episodes of SH	Educational attainment beyond primary level	2.82 (1.25– 6.38)	0.013
		ACE DD genotype	2.35 (1.13–1.53)	0.006
		ACE-I use	1.77 (0.99 –3.13)	0.052
67/men and women		**Frequency**	**Incidence rate ratio (95% CI)**	**p value**
		Logit model		
		Time on insulin (increase of 1 yr)	0.34 (0.18–0.66)	0.001
		eGFR _ 60 ml/min per 1.73m2	0.18 (0.06–0.50)	0.001
		Peripheral neuropathy	0.18 (0.06–0.49)	0.001
		Educational attainment beyond primary school level	0.17 (0.04–0.87)	0.033
		Count model		
		HbA1c (increase of 1%)	1.36 (1.08 –1.71)	0.009
		FSG (increase of 1 mmol/liter)	0.83 (0.73 – 0.94)	0.004
		ACE DD genotype	1.80 (1.00 –3.24)	0.050
Duran-Nah, 2008[104]	Case control	**Variable**	**OR (95% CI)**	**p value**
		Age (years)	0.95 (0.88–0.09)	0.008
Mexico	Multivariate	Diabetes duration (years)	1.110 (1.05–1.2)	0.001
		Illiteracy-primary	3.7 (1.4–10.0)	0.009
NR	Blood glucose < or equal to 72 in presence of neurological clinical picture consistent with a severely confused mental state or worse, non-arousable, should respond to IV glucose	Attending physician (FP)	2.8 (1.02–7.9)	0.04
		Chronic renal failure (yes)	3.0 (1.2–7.7)	0.01
59/men and women		Missed meals (yes)	19.8 (9.1–43.1)	<0.001
		Previous hypoglycemia (yes)	2.9 (1.3–6.5)	0.01
		Combined therapy (yes)	5.2 (2.3–11.8)	<0.01
	92 (cases) patients with hypoglycemia and 188 without (controls)	Polypharmacy use (yes)	4.9 (0.7–35.1)	0.11

Study Location Funding Age/Sex	Study Design Analysis Definition of Severe # of Patients	Risk Factors for Severe Hypoglycemia OR Patient Characteristics If No Formal Risk Factor Analysis		
		Characteristic	OHAs	Insulin	p value
Fadini, 2009[95]	Retrospective Cohort	Age, years	79.7 (11.4)	74.7 (10.1)	0.009
Italy	Unadjusted	Male sex (%)	46.0	41.3	0.66
		Institutionalized (%)	7.9	4.8	0.73
NR	Hypoglycemia that led to hospitalization	First blood glucose (mg/dl)	38.2 (11.2)	39.7 (11.5)	0.33
		Coma (%)	54.0	30.2	0.002
77/men and women		Fall (%)	25.4	17.5	0.27
	126 episodes (63 OHA, 63 Insulin)	Duration of hypoglycemia (h)	8.1 (8.9)	3.9 (4.3)	0.001
		HbA1c (%)	6.75 (1.0)	8.1 (2.1)	<0.001
	Precipitating events: low carb intake without change in therapy n=71, errors in administration of insulin n=19	Serum creatinine (mmol/l)	106.6 (45.4)	120.6 (115.9)	0.64
		eGFR >60 ml/min/1.73 m2	37	43	0.63
		eGFR 30–59 ml/min/m2	21	16	0.32
		eGFR 15–29 ml/min/m2	5	1	0.09
	No association with other typical risk factors (such as education)	eGFR <ml/min/m2	0	3	0.08
		0–4 years from diagnosis(%)	39.7	26.9	0.13
		5–9 years from diagnosis (%)	17.5	9.5	0.19
	In-hospital outcomes: Acute coronary syndrome 17.5% OHA, 19.0% Insulin, p=0.85	10–19 years from diagnosis (%)	17.4	19.1	0.82
		20+ years from diagnosis (%)	25.4	44.5	0.03
		Obesity (%)	30.2	23.8	0.27
		Dyslipidemia (%)	19.0	12.7	0.74
		Hypertension (%)	79.4	79.4	0.78
	Duration of stay 9.8 days OHA, 8.0 days Insulin, p=0.05	Coronary artery disease (%)	39.7	31.7	0.53
		Peripheral artery disease (%)	47.6	38.1	0.27
		Retinopathy (%)	9.5	27.0	0.007
		Known neuropathy (%)	6.3	17.5	0.023
	Death at follow-up 31.7% OHA, 52.4% Insulin p=0.02	Liver disease (%)	3.2	25.4	0.001
		Cancer (%)	12.7	22.2	0.25
		COPD (%)	22.2	11.1	0.19
		Rheumatoid arthritis (%)	0.0	3.2	0.25
		Dementia (%)	3.2	4.8	0.44
		Beta-blockers (%) (selective (%))	19.0 (19.0)	15.9 (12.7)	0.56
		ACE inhibitors (%)	58.7	61.9	0.52
		Aspirin (%)	57.1	41.3	0.46
		NSAIDs (%)	1.6	3.2	0.41
		Cimetidine (%)	0.0	1.6	0.25
		CNS depressants (%)	15.9	17.5	0.49

Study Location Funding Age/Sex	Study Design Analysis Definition of Severe # of Patients	Risk Factors for Severe Hypoglycemia OR Patient Characteristics If No Formal Risk Factor Analysis		
Henderson, 2003[76] Scotland NR 68/men and women	Cross-sectional Unadjusted Required external assistance, symptoms suggestive of hypoglycemia that had resolved following treatment with oral carbohydrate, or had required treatment with parenteral glucose or glucagon 215 interviews, 60 episodes by 32 people 0.28 episodes per patient per year	Frequency of severe hypoglycemia increased with: Age (p<0.05 r=0.2) Duration of diabetes (p<0.05, r=0.2) Duration of insulin therapy (p<0.05, r=0.2) Impaired awareness (9 fold higher rate) – not associated with age duration of DM, or duration of tx with DM Normal awareness: 0.22 episodes/patient/year Impaired awareness 2.15 episodes/patient/year No association with: Lower HbA1c Higher insulin dose		
Hepburn, 1992[99] Scotland NR 63/men and women	Cross-sectional Unadjusted Episode during which the patient was unable to take appropriate restorative action and required the assistance of another person for treatment (either at home or in the hospital) to administer either oral or parenteral glucose, or glucagon by injection 104 type 2 DM patients	r=0.39 (p<0.001) - # episodes and duration of insulin All patients with partial awareness (n=6) and 3 of 80 (4%) with normal awareness had severe hypoglycemia in past year		
		Characteristic	No Severe Hypoglycemia (n=62)	Severe hypoglycemia (n=25)
		Age (years)	62 ± 8	64 ± 11
		Body mass index	28 ± 5	26 ± 4
		Duration of diabetes (yrs)	11	13
		Duration of insulin therapy (yrs)	2	6
		Daily insulin dose (U/kg)	0.6	0.7
		Glycated hemoglobin (%)	10.4	10.7
Holman, 2009[43] **Treat to Target in Type 2 DM (4-T)** UK Industry 62/men and women	RCT Third party assistance needed 708 patients	Hypoglycemic events (no/patient/year)	Biphasic	Prandial	Basal
		All patients			
		Grade 3	0	0	0
		Patients with an HbA1c of less than or equal to 6.5%			
		Grade 3	0	0	0

Risk Factors for Severe Hypoglycemia OR Patient Characteristics If No Formal Risk Factor Analysis

Study / Location / Funding / Age/Sex	Study Design / Analysis / Definition of Severe / # of Patients
Holstein, 2009[102] Germany NR 78/men and women	Case Control; Multivariate; A symptomatic event requiring treatment with IV glucose and confirmed with a BG of <50 mg/dl (<2.8 mmol/l); 43/97 had severe hypoglycemia All on sulfonylurea and no insulin

Characteristic	Control (n=54)	Severe Hypoglycemia (n=43)	p value
Sex (male / female)	28 / 26	20 / 23	0.60 *
Age (years)	80.1 ± 8.8	75.2 ± 10.4	0.01
BMI (kg / m 2)	26.80 ± 4.73	26.72 ± 4.67	0.94
Creatinine (mg/ dl)	1.83 ± 1.23	1.53 ± 0.93	0.18
Creatinine clearance (ml / min)	38.89 ± 18.85	48.91 ± 23.65	0.02
HbA 1c (%)	7.15 ± 0.96	6.73 ± 1.28	0.07
Age at onset of diabetes (years)	69.1 ± 12.3	66.1 ± 14.3	0.30
Diabetes duration (years)	10.8 ± 8.1	8.6 ± 11.3	0.30
Co-medication (number of all drugs)	7 ± 2	6 ± 3	0.08
Metformin treatment (number of patients)	22	13	0.28 *

Variable	Univariate analysis OR and p value	Multivariate analysis and p value
Gender	0.81 (0.36 – 1.80) 0.60	0.79 (0.30 – 2.07) 0.63
Age (years)	0.95 (0.91 – 0.99) 0.02	0.92 (0.88 – 0.98) 0.005
Diabetes duration (years)	0.97 (0.93 – 1.03) 0.31	0.96 (0.91 – 1.01) 0.11
Sulfonylurea daily dose (mg)	1.16 (0.99 – 1.36) 0.07	1.25 (1.03 – 1.52) 0.02
HbA 1c (%)	0.69 (0.45 – 1.04) 0.08	0.67 (0.42 – 1.05) 0.08
KCNJ11 (E23K)	0.54 (0.30 – 0.98) 0.04	0.68 (0.34 – 1.35) 0.27

Study / Location / Funding / Age/Sex	Study Design / Analysis / Definition of Severe / # of Patients
Holstein, 2003[107] 3 countries NR 78/men and women	Case series; Unadjusted; A symptomatic event requiring administration of IV glucose or glucagon; 93 episodes, 37 on glimepiride, 56 on glibenclamide

	Glimepiride (n=37)	Glibenclamide (n=56)	Treatment Differences (95% CI)	p value
Age (years)	77.1±11.2 (43–93)	78.1±9.6 (43–97)	-1.0 (-6.0; 4.0)	0.721
Female sex (%)	57% (21/37)	61% (34/56)	-4.0% (-24.4; 16.5)	0.830
Body mass index	24.6±4.5 (16.9–38.4)	24.8±4.5 (17.8–36.9)	-0.2 (-2.6; 2.2)	0.942
Duration of diabetes (years)	7.0±7.0 (0–32)	10.5±8.7 (0–33)	-3.5 (-7.4; 0.4)	0.095
HbA1c (HPLC; non-diabetic range 3.4–4.9%)	5.4±0.7 (4.6–7.7)	5.2±0.9 (3.7–7.5)	0.2 (-0.2; 0.6)	0.345
Initial blood glucose (mmol/l)	1.9±0.66 (0.78–2.9)	1.8±0.89 (0–3.7)	0.1 (-0.24; 0.6)	0.443
Co-medication (number of drugs)	6.2±3.0 (0–15)	3.6±3.0 (0–16)	2.60 (1.2; 4.0)	<0.001
Creatinine-clearance (ml/min)	38±23 (10–87)	54±32 (8–180)	-16.0 (-30.1; -1.9)	0.016

Possible causes identified for 75 of 93 (81%): missed meals (59%), alcohol (15%), increased activity (5%), incorrect dosing (1%)

Study Location Funding Age/Sex	Study Design Analysis Definition of Severe # of Patients	Risk Factors for Severe Hypoglycemia OR Patient Characteristics If No Formal Risk Factor Analysis					
Holstein, 2003[109] Germany Industry 84/men and women	Case series A symptomatic event requiring an IV glucose or glucagon injection that relieved symptoms and was confirmed by blood glucose measurement 30,768 patients in ED, 264 cases of SH Rate 1.5 episodes per 100 patients in insulin treated DM2 0.4 episodes per 100 for overall DM2	Characteristic in type 2 DM (n=148) with SH Age (year) 76 +/- 12 (44-95) Percent female 64% (95/148) BMI 25.7 +/- 4.8 (15.8-39.7) Initial blood glucose (mg/dl) 34 +/- 16 (0-61) Diabetes duration 17 +/- 11 (0-40) HbA1c% 6.2 +/- 1.8 (3.9-15.5) Renal failure (cr clearance less than 60 ml/min) 54% (80/148) Comorbidity (number of concomitant diseases 3.6 +/- 2.6 (0-7) Comedication (number of drugs) 3.3 +/- 3.0 (0-18) Patients with recurrent hypoglycemia in the study period 12% (14/121)					
		Characteristic	CT (n=78)	SU (n=45)	CT+SU (n=25)	pvalue CT vs SU	pvalue CT vs CT+SU	pvalue SU vs CT+SU
		Age (year)	76 +/- 11	79 +/- 13	72 +/- 10	0.176	0.109	0.023
		Percent female	63%	62%	44%	1.000	0.109	0.209
		BMI	25.0 +/- 5.1	24.4 +/- 5.0	24.4 +/- 3.3			
		Diabetes duration (years)						
		Initial blood glucose	19+/-10	12+/-10	16+/-10	<0.001	0.195	0.113
		HbA1c %	38+/-19	31+/-16	34+/-16	0.040	0.345	0.455
		Insulin dose	6.7+/-2.0	5.4+/-0.9	6.6+/-1.8	<0.001	0.824	<0.001
			37+/-18		27+/-20		0.017	
		Frequency and dose of glibenclamide		n=38, 6.1+/- 3.1	n=18, 7.2+/-1.1			
		Frequency and dose of glimepiride		n=6, 2.5+/-0.8	n=7 2.1+/-0.6			
		Comedication (number of drugs)	3.7 +/- 2.5	3.8 +/- 2.8	5.2 +/- 3.6	0.838	0.022	0.075
		Renal failure (cr cl < 60 ml/min)	53% (41/78)	58% (26/45)	52% (13/25)	0.707	1.000	0.802
		Attributed causes for 68/148 (46%) episodes in type 2 patients: missed meals (59%), incorrect dosing (19%), alcohol (13%), increased activity (9%)						

Study Location Funding Age/Sex	Study Design Analysis Definition of Severe # of Patients	Risk Factors for Severe Hypoglycemia OR Patient Characteristics If No Formal Risk Factor Analysis
Holstein, 2011[103] Germany NR 77/men and women	Case control Multivariate Symptomatic event requiring treatment with IV glucose and was confirmed by BG <50 mg/dl 102 cases of SH, 101 controls	(see detail below)

Basic characteristics of type 2 diabetic patients with sulfonylurea-induced hypoglycemia versus control group

Variable	Severe hypoglycemia (n = 102)	Control (n = 101)	p value
Sex (female/male)	45/57	51/50	0.36
Age (years)	77.4 ± 9.2	79.3±9.2	0.13
Body mass index (kg/m2)	26.7±5.5	27.0±4.4	0.76
Serum creatinine (mg/dl)	1.55±0,87	1.72±1.03	0.19
Creatinine clearance (ml/min)	45.8±22.6	38.0±18.1	0.02
HbA1c (%)	6.5±1.2	7.2±1.3	0.0004
Co-medication (number of drugs)	7.0±2.8	7.4±2.8	0.28
Duration of diabetes (years)	11.0±9.9	11.5±8.3	0.71

Patients with glimepiride mean daily dose 76 (74.5%) 2.8±1.6 mg   81 (80.2%) 2.3±1.3 mg   0.33 (chi2) 0.04 (t-test)

Patients with glibenclamide mean daily dose 25 (24.5%) 6.1±3.7 mg   18 (17.8%) 5.0±3.6 mg   0.2 (chi2) 0.3 (t-test)

Patients with gliquidone mean daily dose 1 (1.0%) 30 mg   2 (2%) 60 mg   0.62

Additional treatment with metformin mean daily dose 37 (36%) 1731±602 mg   43 (43%) 1715±494 mg   0.36 (chi2) 0.90 (t-test)

Additional treatment with insulin mean daily dose 29 (28%) 36.4±22 I.E. 20 (20%) 36.8±21.5 I.E.   0.15 (chi2) 0.96 (t-test)

Co-medication with other CYP2C9 main substrates 24 (24%) 33 (49%)   0.001 (chi2)

Co-medication with other drugs being at least one CYP2C9 substrate 39 (39%) 32 (47%)   0.30 (chi2)

Risk factors for severe hypoglycemia in 102 sulfonylurea-treated type 2 diabetic patients with severe hypoglycemia versus control group (n=101)

Variable	Relative risk (95% CI)	p value
HbA1c (%)	1.56 (1.20–2.04)	0.001
Dose of sulfonylurea	1.00 (0.96–1.04)	0.95
CYP2C9-genotypes *2/*2, *2/*3, and *3/*3	0.58 (0.14–2.50)	0.47
Co-medication with other CYP2C9-main substrates	0.34 (0.17–0.65)	0.001
Co-medication with other drugs being at least one CYP2C9-substrate	0.72 (0.39–1.34)	0.30
Co-medication with insulin	1.61 (0.84–3.09)	0.15
Co-medication with angiotensin-converting enzyme inhibitor	1.35 (0.77–2.34)	0.29
Co-medication with analgetics	1.21 (0.59–2.50)	0.60
Co-medication with gyrase inhibitors	0.99 (0.20–5.03)	0.99
Presence of coronary heart disease	2.38 (1.35–4.18)	0.003
Presence of heart failure	1.46 (0.84–2.55)	0.18
Presence of dementia	1.97 (0.94–4.15)	0.09
Previous participation at structured diabetes education	1.09 (0.59–2.00)	0.79
Kind of accommodation (home vs. nursing home)	1.29 (0.87–1.92)	0.21

Study Location Funding Age/Sex	Study Design Analysis Definition of Severe # of Patients	Risk Factors for Severe Hypoglycemia OR Patient Characteristics If No Formal Risk Factor Analysis			
Holstein, 2001[17]	Prospective cohort	Basic characteristics of the diabetic patients presenting with sulfonylurea-induced hypoglycemia			
Same data set as Holstein 2003 Germany above	Unadjusted	Characteristic	Glibenclamide +glimepiride (n=1)	Glibenclamide (n=38)	Glimepiride (n=6)	Treatment difference and 95% CI glibenclamide vs glimepiride

Characteristic	Glibenclamide +glimepiride (n=1)	Glibenclamide (n=38)	Glimepiride (n=6)	Treatment difference and 95% CI glibenclamide vs glimepiride
Age (years)	84	83.5	83.5	0 (-17.1; 9.1)
Sex (% female)	0%	63.2%	66.7%	-3.5 (-44.1; 37.3)
Diabetes duration (years)	4	6.0	16.0	-10 (-19.0; 0.8)
BMI (kg/m²)	24.8	22.9	28.2	-5.3 (-10.7; 1.1)
Sulfonylurea dose (mg)	3.5 and 2	4.4	3.0	1.4 (0.6; 6.6)
Initial venous blood glucose (mmol/l)	2.24	1.7	1.8	-0.1 (-0.97; 0.95)
HbA1c (HPLC; non-diabetic range 3.4–4.9%)	5.6	5.25	4.7	0.55 (-0.3; 1.9)
Patients with impaired renal function	1/1 (100%)	23/38 (60.5%)	4/6 (66.7%)	-6.1% (-46.9; 34.7)
Co-medication (number of drugs)	7	3.0	3.5	-0.5 (-3.7; 3.1)
Participation in diabetes education programs (%)	0%	3% (1/38)	0%	Not done

Holstein, 2001[17]: A symptomatic event requiring an IV glucose or glucagon injection that relieved symptoms and was confirmed by blood glucose measurement. 30,768 patients in ED, 264 cases of SH. Rate 1.5 episodes per 100 patients in insulin treated DM2. 0.4 episodes per 100 for overall DM2.

Germany / Industry / 84/men and women

Study Location Funding Age/Sex	Study Design Analysis Definition of Severe # of Patients	Risk Factors for Severe Hypoglycemia OR Patient Characteristics If No Formal Risk Factor Analysis
HTN in DM study IV, 1996[91]	RCT	No difference between allocations in the proportion of patients having hypoglycemic episodes

HTN in DM study IV, 1996[91]: Unadjusted. Major hypoglycemic events: requiring medical assistance or hospitalization. 758 patients. UK / Government/Industry / 57/men and women.

Annual rates of major hypoglycemic episodes over 5 years

Time post randomization	Captopril	Atenolol	Less tight control
n	247	223	228
1st year	2.5%	0.5%	0.8%
2nd year	0.9%	1.0%	0.4%
3rd year	0	1.0%	0.8%
4th year	1.0%	3.1%	0.9%
5th year	0.5%	1.6%	1.8%
Ever over 5 years	4.0%	4.9%	3.1%

Leese, 2003[25]: Retrospective cohort. No adjustment. Any episode requiring external help. 7,678 with type 2 DM. DART/MEMO. Scotland / Industry / 65/men and women.

	Number	Age (years)	HbA1c %	Duration of DM (years)	BMI	Sex (% male)
On insulin, no hypo	835	63.2	8.23	11.8	30.1	47.7
On insulin, hypo	66	66.6	7.87	13.5	26.7	47.0
P value		0.038	0.097	0.137	<0.001	0.914
On sulfonylurea, no hypo	2,800	65.4	7.16	6.3	29.6	52.2
On sulfonylurea, hypo	23	65.0	8.00	7.2	28.1	47.8
P value		0.884	0.064	0.517	0.122	0.687

Study / Location / Funding / Age/Sex	Study Design / Analysis / Definition of Severe / # of Patients	Risk Factors for Severe Hypoglycemia OR Patient Characteristics If No Formal Risk Factor Analysis	HR (95% CI)	p value
Miller, 2010[89] ACCORD data	RCT	*HMA (both intensive and standard arms)*		
2 countries	Multivariate adjusted	Female (v male)	1.21 (1.02 to 1.43)	0.0300
Government and industry	Episodes of hypoglycemia requiring emergency care or be admitted to a hospital: Hypoglycemia requiring medical assistance (HMA), or "low blood glucose" requiring any assistance, medical or non medical (HA), after March 2003: plasma glucose of less than 2.8 mmol/l (50 mg/dl) or symptoms that promptly resolved with carbohydrate also a requirement	Race		<0.0001
62/men and women		Non Hispanic white	1.0	
		African-American	1.43 (1.20 to 1.71)	<0.0001
		Hispanic	0.93 (0.68 to 1.27)	0.6500
		Other	0.64 (0.47 to 0.88)	0.0100
		History of CV disease (yes v no)	1.10 (0.94 to 1.28)	0.2200
		History of peripheral neuropathy (yes v no)	1.19 (1.02 to 1.38)	0.0300
		Time since diagnosis of diabetes (years)		0.7394
		< or equal to 5	1.0	
		6-10	0.98 (0.77 to 1.24)	0.8500
		11-15	1.06 (0.83 to 1.37)	0.6200
		16+	1.37 (1.09 to 1.73)	0.0100
		BMI		0.0023
		<25	1.0	
		>or equal to 25 to< 30	0.78 (0.60 to 1.02)	0.0700
		30+	0.65 (0.50 to 0.85)	<0.0001
		Albumin to creatinine ratio		<0.0001
		<30	1.0	
		30-300	1.20 (1.02 to 1.43)	0.0300
		>300	1.74 (1.37 to 2.21)	<0.0001
		Serum creatinine (micromol/l)		0.0010
		<88.4	1.0	
		88.4-114.9	1.21 (1.02 to 1.43)	0.0300
		>114.9	1.66 (1.25 to 2.19)	<0.0001
		Age (per 1 year increase)	1.03 (1.02 to 1.05)	<0.0001

Study / Location / Funding / Age/Sex	Study Design / Analysis / Definition of Severe / # of Patients	Risk Factors for Severe Hypoglycemia OR Patient Characteristics If No Formal Risk Factor Analysis
Miller, 2001[100]	Cross-sectional	**No significant predictors of severe hypoglycemia**
United States	Multivariate	Age, sex, race, diabetes duration, BMI, follow-up fasting plasma glucose level, follow-up HbA1c level, type of diabetes therapy, hypoglycemia at baseline visit, and whether diabetes medication therapy was increased at the baseline visit
Government	Loss of consciousness or other major alteration of mental status caused by hypoglycemia that required the assistance of another person to treat the condition	
70/men and women	5/1055	

Patient Number	Sex/Age, y	BMI	Diabetes Duration, y	HbA1c, %	Therapy Type	Insulin Dosage, U/kg per day
1	F/73.7	48.1	18.7	6.3	Insulin	0.32
2	F/53.2	29.6	6.4	5.6	Insulin and metformin	0.63
3	M/68.1	34.9	18.4	8.3	Insulin	0.51
4	F/74.2	26.6	23.3	8.3	Insulin	0.44
5	M/61.5	N/A	16.4	12.1	Insulin	0.32

All black race

Predictors and Consequences of Severe Hypoglycemia in Adults with Diabetes – Systematic Review of the Evidence

Risk Factors for Severe Hypoglycemia OR Patient Characteristics If No Formal Risk Factor Analysis

Study Location Funding Age/Sex	Study Design Analysis Definition of Severe # of Patients		Cases, % (n 1339)	Controls, % (n 13,390)	Crude OR (95% CI)	Adjusted OR*(95% CI)
Quilliam, 2011[27]	Nested case control	Independent predictors of inpatient hypoglycemia admissions.				
Marketscan Database	Multivariate	Variable				
United States	Hypoglycemia requiring hospitalization, used ICD9 codes	Gender				
		Female	49.2	46.3	1.00 (N/A)	1.00 (N/A)
Industry	1339 cases, 13,390 controls	Male	50.8	53.7	0.89 (0.80–0.99)	0.84 (0.73–0.96)
		Age, y				
55/men and women		18–34	1.3	2.1	1.00 (N/A)	1.00 (N/A)
		35–49	13.3	21.1	0.99 (0.60–1.63)	1.01 (0.58–1.79)
		50–64	82.6	74.5	1.75 (1.08–2.84)	1.14 (0.66–1.97)
		_65	2.8	2.4	1.88 (1.04–3.39)	0.91 (0.46–1.81)
		Oral diabetes medications†,‡				
		Sulfonylureas: Continuous availability§	41.1	30.0	2.36 (2.06–2.70)	2.25 (1.93–2.63)
		Sulfonylureas: Intermittent availability	25.1	14.6	2.88 (2.48–3.35)	2.28 (1.90–2.74)
		Metformin: Continuous availability§	34.1	47.9	0.48 (0.42–0.55)	0.62 (0.53–0.73)
		Metformin: Intermittent availability	23.8	23.3	0.70 (0.60–0.81)	0.76 (0.64–0.92)
		Thiazolidinediones: Continuous availability§	22.9	23.8	1.00 (0.87–1.15)	1.06 (0.90–1.24)
		Thiazolidinediones: Intermittent availability	16.9	13.8	1.27 (1.09–1.49)	1.22 (1.01–1.47)
		Other OHA: Continuous availability§	4.5	3.9	1.15 (0.88–1.52)	1.11 (0.80–1.55)
		Other OHA: Intermittent availability	3.7	3.2	1.17 (0.86–1.59)	1.09 (0.75–1.59)

Study Location Funding Age/Sex Study Design Analysis Definition of Severe # of Patients	Risk Factors for Severe Hypoglycemia OR Patient Characteristics If No Formal Risk Factor Analysis	Cases, % (n 1339)	Controls, % (n 13,390)	Crude OR (95% CI)	Adjusted OR*(95% CI)
Quilliam, 2011[27]					
Continued	Other medications#				
	Allopurinol	5.5	2.6	2.15 (1.66–2.78)	1.54 (1.13–2.12)
	Benzodiazepine	14.6	6.2	2.57 (2.17–3.03)	1.90 (1.55–2.33)
	Beta-blocker	35.1	21.3	2.01 (1.78–2.26)	1.20 (1.03–1.40)
	Blood glucose monitoring supplies	30.9	30.6	1.02 (0.90–1.15)	0.83 (0.71–0.96)
	Fluoroquinolone	10.7	2.5	4.69 (3.82–5.77)	2.59 (1.99–3.39)
	Insulin	16.8	6.7	2.84 (2.42–3.33)	2.23 (1.83–2.72)
	NSAID	13.8	10.4	1.38 (1.17–1.63)	1.27 (1.05–1.54)
	Trimethoprim	3.3	0.9	3.81 (2.68–5.41)	1.97 (1.26–3.08)
	Comorbid conditions				
	Previous outpatient visit for hypoglycemia	12.5	0.9	16.17 (12.60–20.76)	7.88 (5.68–10.93)
	Previous ED visit for hypoglycemia	6.2	0.1	48.53 (28.80–81.78)	9.48 (4.95–18.15)
	Macrovascular complications				
	Arrhythmia	6.8	1.4	5.25 (4.05–6.81)	1.69 (1.17–2.44)
	Coronary artery disease	21.0	7.8	3.12 (2.69–3.61)	1.48 (1.21–1.81)
	Heart failure	14.0	1.5	10.99 (8.86–13.64)	2.33 (1.72–3.15)
	Stroke	3.4	0.4	9.62 (6.37–14.52)	2.78 (1.62–4.77)
	Microvascular complications				
	Acute renal failure	8.3	0.6	15.43 (11.43–20.83)	3.10 (2.05–4.67)
	Chronic renal pathophysiology	8.4	1.1	8.37 (6.49–10.81)	2.22 (1.56–3.15)
	Ulcer	6.4	1.4	4.98 (3.82–6.49)	1.71 (1.20–2.44)
	Charlson comorbidity (per 1 U change)			1.72 (1.66–1.79)	1.37 (1.32–1.44)

*Adjusted for all factors listed in the table.
†As identified in pharmacy claims in the 6 months before the index date.
‡Nonavailability of the medication/class of medication is the referent group.
§Participants with continuous availability had medication coverage in each of all six 30-day periods preceding the index date.
‖Participants with intermittent availability had medication coverage in at least 1 of the preceding 6 intervals.
¶Includes persons taking glucosidase inhibitors, dipeptidyl peptidase-4 inhibitors, or meglitinides.
#Defined as medication availability in the previous 30 days.

Study Location Funding Age/Sex	Study Design Analysis Definition of Severe # of Patients	Risk Factors for Severe Hypoglycemia OR Patient Characteristics If No Formal Risk Factor Analysis
Sarkar, 2010[78] United States Government 58/men and women	Cross-sectional Multivariate Answer yes to the question ""In the past year, how many times have you had a SEVERE low blood sugar reaction, such as passing out or needing help to treat the reaction?" 14,357 surveys included, 1,579 reported significant hypoglycemia	Self reported Health literacy

Risk Factors detail (Sarkar):

	unadjusted OR (95% CI)	adjusted OR (95% CI)
Problems learning	1.5 (1.3-1.8)	1.4 (1.1-1.7)
Need help reading	1.5 (1.3-1.8)	1.3 (1.1-1.6)
Not confident with forms	1.5 (1.3-1.8)	1.3 (1.1-1.6)

p value for all <0.0001

Study Location Funding Age/Sex	Study Design Analysis Definition of Severe # of Patients	Risk Factors
Sato, 2010[106] Japan NR 75/men and women	Case control study Unadjusted Stratified by age, sex, HbA1c, duration of diabetes, and medications Characteristic symptoms and a plasma glucose level of than 50 mg/dl, which required IV glucose 32 cases, 125 controls	Clinical characteristics of patients with or without severe hypoglycemia.

Variable	Severe hypoglycemic group (n = 32)	Diabetic control group (n = 125)	p-value
Age	74.8 ± 8.5	63.7 ± 11.3	<0.001†
Sex (M/F)	12 (37%)/20 (63%)	82 (66%)/43 (34%)	<0.001†
BMI (kg/m2)	23.2 ± 4.4	24.2 ± 4.0	0.26
HbA1c‡ (%)	6.54 ± 1.1	8.11 ± 1.5	<0.001†
Creatinine (mg/dl)	0.88 ± 0.55	0.78 ± 0.28	0.69
eGFR§ (ml/min/1.73 m2)	71.0 ± 33.5	77.6 ± 23.0	0.29
Duration of diabetes (year)	14.9 ± 10.2	7.3 ± 5.8	<0.001†
Number of total drugs	6.0 ± 2.6	4.3 ± 2.6	0.001†
Dosage of sulfonylurea			
Glimepiride (mg/day)	2.7 ± 1.7	1.2 ± 0.93	<0.001†
Glibenclamide (mg/day)	4.25 ± 2.5	4.27 ± 2.3	0.88
Comedication			
Metformin	9 (28%)	45 (36%)	0.4
Pioglitazone	7 (22%)	16 (13%)	0.16
a-glucosidase inhibitor	16 (50%)	27 (22%)	0.001†
Insulin	6 (17%)	18 (14%)	0.36

Data are expressed as mean ± standard deviation or %.
†Significant difference (p < 0.05).
‡At the time of the event of severe hypoglycemia in the hypoglycemic group.
§eGFR calculated according to the Modification of Diet in Renal Disease Study equation.
eGFR: Estimated glomerular filtration rate; F: Female; HbA1c: Hemoglobin A1c; M: Male.

Study Location Funding Age/Sex	Study Design Analysis Definition of Severe # of Patients	Risk Factors for Severe Hypoglycemia OR Patient Characteristics If No Formal Risk Factor Analysis			
Shen, 2008[101]	Cross Sectional	Acute hypoglycemic condition			
United States	Multivariate		Odds ratio (95% CI)		
NR	ICD-9-CM code for hypoglycemia, patients had to be admitted to hospital	African American	1.62 (1.55-1.69)		
		Hispanic	1.24 (1.18-1.30)		
66/men and women	787,836 discharges	Asian	1.15 (1.03-1.75)		
Shorr, 1997[97]	Retrospective cohort	Covariate	Person Years	No. of events	Rate	Relative Risk (95% CI)
United States	Multivariate	Drug				
		Sulfonylurea	20714	255	1.23	reference value
Government	Hospitalization, emergency department admission, or death	Insulin	11978	331	2.76	2.1 (1.8-2.5)
		Insulin and sulfonylurea	355	12	3.38	2.9 (1.6-9.2)
65 and older/ men and women	associated with hypoglycemic symptoms and a blood glucose of less than 2.8 mmol/l (50 mg/dl)	Age, y				
		65-69	10627	156	1.46	reference value
		70-74	8281	130	1.57	1.1 (0.9-1.4)
		75-79	7159	142	1.98	1.5 (1.2-1.9)
	586 persons with severe	>80	6980	170	2.43	1.8 (1.4-2.3)
	hypoglycemia out of 33048 person	Sex				
	years	M	5304	107	2.01	reference value
		F	27743	491	1.77	0.8 (0.7-1.0)
		Race				
		W	21207	313	1.47	reference value
		B	8974	239	2.66	2.0 (1.7-2.4)
		County of residence				
		Rural (non-SMSA)	9121	198	2.17	reference value
		Rural (SMSA)	7169	137	1.91	1.1 (0.8-1.3)
		Urban	16758	263	1.57	0.9 (0.7-1.1)
		Days since hospital discharge				
		>366	21491	272	1.27	reference value
		31-365	10096	231	2.29	1.7 (1.4-2.0)
		1-30	1460	95	6.50	4.5 (3.5-5.7)
		Nursing home resident				
		No	26233	444	1.69	reference value
		Yes	6815	154	2.26	1.0 (0.8-1.3)
		No. of concomitant medications				
		0-4	24440	395	1.61	reference value
		>5	8608	203	2.35	1.3 (1.1-1.5)
		New hypoglycemic drug therapy				
		No	31808	559	1.75	reference value
		Yes	1240	39	3.15	1.4 (1.0-1.9)

Study Location Funding Age/Sex	Study Design Analysis Definition of Severe # of Patients	Risk Factors for Severe Hypoglycemia OR Patient Characteristics If No Formal Risk Factor Analysis		
Sotiropoulos, 2005[108]	Case series	Out of 207 patients with severe hypoglycemia		
		Characterisitic	**Mean (SD)**	**Range**
Greece	No comparison group or risk factor adjustment	Age (years)	62.1 (8.7)	45–88
		Duration of diabetes (years)	7.4 (2.8)	1–14
NR	Comatose or pre-comatose status (according to the Glasgow coma scale) on arrival at the emergency ward, serum glucose level < 2.8 mmol/l, and necessity for IV glucose administration for resuscitation	HbA1c level (%)	6.8 (1.3)	
		Characteristic	**No.**	**%**
62/men and women		Sex		
		Male	85	41.1
		Female	122	58.9
		Presentation		
		Coma	146	70.5
		Semi-coma	61	29.5
	2858 patients admitted, 207 had severe hypoglycemia (7.2%)	Usual treatment		
		Insulin	72	34.8
		Sulfonylureas	132	63.8
		Insulin and sulfonylureas	3	1.4
		Follow-up in diabetes clinic		
		Yes	59	28.5
		No	148	71.5
		Educational status		
		Illiterate	28	13.5
		Elementary	117	56.5
		Middle	47	22.7
		Higher	15	7.3
		Diabetes knowledge		
		Poor	175	85.4
		Good	30	14.6
		Causes of hypoglycaemia		
		Missed meal	76	30.8
		Chronic renal failure	54	21.9
		Exercise	28	11.4
		Alcohol	20	8.2
		Dosage error	16	6.5
		Unknown	34	13.9

Predictors and Consequences of Severe Hypoglycemia
in Adults with Diabetes – Systematic Review of the Evidence

Study Location Funding Age/Sex	Study Design Analysis Definition of Severe # of Patients	Risk Factors for Severe Hypoglycemia OR Patient Characteristics If No Formal Risk Factor Analysis
Stepka, 1993[98]	Retrospective cohort	Serum creatinine >2 mg/dL prior to hypoglycemia: (20) 20.2% of insulin treated, (1) 2.7% of oral med group
		Ischemic heart disease: (56) 55.5% of insulin group, (28) 80% of oral med group
Poland	No adjustment	Leg vessel disease: (29) 28.7% of insulin group, (17) 48.6% of oral med group
		Polyneuropathy: (17) 16.8% of insulin group, (3) 8% of oral med group
NR	Requiring immediate aid in a health care institution	Retinopathy: (16) 15.8% of insulin group, (3) 8% or oral med group
66/men and women	20,978 admissions	Causes (allowing for multiple causes)
		Physical effort: (13) 12.9% insulin, (6) 17.1% oral meds
		Dietary Non-compliance: (60) 59.4% insulin, (14) 40% oral meds
	101 DM2 treated with insulin	Dosage error: (7) 7% insulin, (4) 11.4% oral meds
	36 DM2 treated with orals	Alcohol: (7) 7% insulin, (2) 5.7% oral meds
	10 DM3 (secondary DM)	Unknown: (12)11.9% insulin, (7) 20% oral meds
Sugarman, 1991[96]	Retrospective cohort	46.8% of admissions were males
		9.5% had change in prescribe dose of hypoglycemic agent within 30 days prior to admission
United States	Stratified by age	
	Required admission to the hospital for hypoglycemia for NIDDM	RR=2.79 (95%CI 1.6-4.9) (risk of hospitalization if prescribed glyburide vs. chlorpropamide)
NR		
65/men and women	126 hypoglycemia associated admissions	
	4.7 per 1000 person years	

138

Study Location Funding Age/Sex	Study Design Analysis Definition of Severe # of Patients	Risk Factors for Severe Hypoglycemia OR Patient Characteristics If No Formal Risk Factor Analysis	No. (%) Hypoglycemia (n=1465)	Nonhypoglycemia (n=15,202)	p value
Whitmer, 2009[94]	Longitudinal Cohort	Age at survey, mean(SD), y	66.32 (7.54)	64.78 (7)	<0.001
	Unadjusted	Education[d]			0.09
Kaiser Permanente Northern California Diabetes Registry	Hospitalization and ED diagnoses of hypoglycemia using codes 251.0, 251.1, and 251.2	Elementary or grade school	108 (7.4)	1004 (6.6)	
		High/trade/business school	607 (41.4)	5997 (39.3)	
		College/higher degree	750 (51.2)	8222 (54.1)	
	16,667 patients	Men	804 (54.9)	8289 (54.5)	0.79
	1465 with hypoglycemia	Race/ethnicity			<0.001
United States		White	877 (59.8)	9588 (63.1)	
		African American	261 (17.8)	1626 (10.7)	
Government		Hispanic	159 (10.8)	1667 (10.9)	
		Asian	125 (8.5)	1917 (12.6)	
65/men and women		Native American	39 (2.6)	341 (2.2)	
		Other	4 (0.3)	63 (0.4)	
		Duration of diabetes from self report in 1994, mean (SD), y	13.72 (9.2)	9.15 (7.9)	
		Duration of Kaiser Permanente membership, mean (SD), y	22.66 (5.32)	22.98 (5.34)	0.03
		Medical utilization rate 2003-2004, mean (SD), y	20.12 (16.60)	15.2 (12.71)	<0.001
		Time since first diabetes diagnosis in Kaiser Permanente system, mean (SD), y	15.24 (3.59)	14.52 (2.89)	<0.001
		Comorbidity			
		Heart disease	1224 (83.5)	9368 (61.6)	<0.001
		Hyperlipidemia	1298 (88.6)	13,488 (88.7)	0.89
		Hypertension	1429 (97.5)	14,557 (95.8)	0.001
		Stroke	645 (43.0)	4389 (28.9)	<0.001
		End-stage renal disease	167 (11.4)	416 (2.74)	<0.001
		HbA1c 1995-2002, mean (SD),%	8.22 (1.29)	8.08 (1.30)	<0.001

Predictors and Consequences of Severe Hypoglycemia in Adults with Diabetes – Systematic Review of the Evidence

Study Location Funding Age/Sex	Study Design Analysis Definition of Severe # of Patients	Risk Factors for Severe Hypoglycemia OR Patient Characteristics If No Formal Risk Factor Analysis		
Whitmer, 2009[94]		**No. (%) Hypoglycemia (n=1465)**	**Nonhypoglycemia (n=15,202)**	**p value**
Continued		Diabetes treatment type 2002-2003		<0.001
		Insulin only		
		533 (37.75)	2157 (14.19)	
		Oral only		
		446 (30.44)	8615 (56.67)	
		Insulin and oral agents		
		352 (24.03)	2794 (18.38)	
		Nonpharmacological-controlled		
		114 (7.70)	1636 (10.70)	
		Years of insulin use from 1994 to censored date, mean number		<0.001
		7.23 (2.6)	6.52 (2.94)	

Frequency of hypoglycemic episodes by dementia status

		Dementia (n=1822) No. (%)	**Nondementia (n=14,845)**	**Age-adjusted incidence rates per 10,000 person-years (95% CI)**	**Excess attributable risk per year, % (95% CI)**
		Any hypoglycemia			
		No			
		1572 (10.34)	13,630 (89.66)	327.60 (311.02-343.18)	
		Yes			
		250 (16.95)	1215 (83.05)[b]	566.82 (496.52-637.48)	2.39 (1.72-3.01)
		No. of hypoglycemic episodes			
		0			
		1572 (10.34)	13,630 (89.66)	327.60 (311.02-343.18)	
		1			
		150 (14.84)	852 (85.16)	491.73 (412.60-570.80)	1.64 (0.91-2.36)
		2			
		57 (22.26)	201 (77.74)	761.75 (561.24-962.27)	4.34 (2.36-6.32)
		3 or more			
		43 (20.40)	162 (79.60)[b]	755.46 (526.46-984.46)	4.28 (2.10-6.44)

[b]p value less than 0.001

Study / Location / Funding / Age/Sex: Zoungas, 2010[90]; ADVANCE data; 20 countries; Government/Industry; 66/men and women

Study Design / Analysis / Definition of Severe / # of Patients: RCT. Univariate and multivariate adjusted Cox proportional regression models. BGL less than 2.8 mmol/l (50 mg/dl) and the presence of typical signs and symptoms of hypoglycemia, transient dysfunction of the CNS who were unable to treat themselves (requiring help from another person)

Risk Factors for Severe Hypoglycemia OR Patient Characteristics If No Formal Risk Factor Analysis

Risk Factor	Unadjusted HR (95% CI)	p value	Adjusted HR (95% CI)	p value
Age (per year)	1.06 (1.04 - 1.08)	<0.0001	1.05 (1.03 - 1.07)	<0.0001
Gender (female vs. male)	1.08 (0.83 - 1.40)	0.56	1.02 (1.00 - 1.04)	0.03
Diabetes duration (per year)	1.05 (1.03 - 1.07)	<0.0001	1.17 (0.89 - 1.54)	0.27
History of Macrovascular disease (yes vs. no)	1.25 (0.96 - 1.64)	0.10	2.14 (1.47 - 3.11)	<0.0001
History of Microvascular disease (yes vs. no)	2.62 (1.92 - 3.57)	<0.0001	1.04 (0.96 - 1.13)	0.35
Glycated hemoglobin (per 1%)	1.08 (1.00 - 1.17)	0.05	1.01 (1.00 - 1.01)	<0.0001
Creatinine level (per µmol/L)	1.01 (1.00 - 1.01)	<0.0001	1.00 (1.00 - 1.00)	0.58
Albumin to Creatinine ratio (per µg/ml)	1.001 (1.00 - 1.002)	<0.01	0.95 (0.93 - 0.98)	<0.01
Body Mass Index (per kg/m2)	0.95 (0.93 - 0.98)	<0.01	1.43 (1.09 - 1.88)	0.01
Ever smoker (yes vs. no)	1.32 (1.02 - 1.71)	0.03	0.98 (0.96 - 1.00)	0.05
Age at completion of formal education (per year)	0.97 (0.95 - 0.99)	<0.01	0.93 (0.87 - 0.99)	0.01
Mini Mental State Examination score (per 1/30)	0.89 (0.84 - 0.93)	<0.0001		
Sulfonylurea alone (yes vs. no)	1.09 (0.81 - 1.46)	0.58		
Metformin alone (yes vs. no)	0.43 (0.27 - 0.69)	<0.001	0.63 (0.36 - 1.09)	0.10
Two or more oral glucose lowering agents (yes vs. no)	1.79 (1.37 - 2.34)	<0.001	1.50 (1.10 - 2.03)	<0.01
Any blood pressure lowering agent (yes vs. no)	0.89 (0.67 - 1.18)	0.42		
Treatment allocation (intensive vs. standard glucose control)	1.86 (1.42 - 2.44)	<0.0001	1.88 (1.42 - 2.48)	<0.001

141

Table 5. Risk Factors for Severe Hypoglycemia Reported in the Individual Studies

Study Year	Age	Gender	Diabetes Duration	A1c	Previous Hypoglycemia	Polypharmacy	Education Level	BMI	Renal Disease	Impaired Awareness	Microvascular Complications	Macrovascular complications	Dementia or psych	Time on insulin	Marital status	Smoking	Intense vs Standard contro	Metformin	Sulfonylurea	Other agents	Insulin or insulin dose	Alcohol	Race	Other
Akram, 2006[84]	✓	✓	✓	✓					✓	✓	✓	✓		✓	✓	✓		✓			✓	✓		✓
Alvarez Guisasola, 2008[85]	✓			✓																				
Asplund, 1991[105]			✓			✓			✓										✓					✓
Bodmer, 2008[24]			✓		✓	✓									✓				✓		✓			
Bruce, 2009[92]	✓	✓	✓	✓	✓		✓	✓	✓		✓	✓							✓		✓			✓
Davis, 2010[16]	✓	✓	✓	✓	✓	✓	✓	✓	✓		✓		✓	✓					✓		✓	✓		✓
Davis, 2011[93]	✓		✓	✓	✓	✓	✓		✓		✓										✓			✓
Duran-Nah, 2008[104]	✓	✓	✓	✓		✓	✓	✓	✓		✓	✓	✓								✓			✓
Fadini, 2009[95]	✓	✓	✓	✓				✓	✓												✓			✓
Henderson, 2003[76]	✓		✓	✓				✓		✓				✓							✓			
Hepburn, 1992[99]	✓		✓	✓				✓		✓				✓							✓			
Holman, 2009[43]	✓			✓					✓			✓						✓	✓		✓			✓
HTN in DM IV, 1996	✓	✓	✓	✓				✓	✓															✓
Holstein, 2001[17]	✓	✓	✓	✓		✓		✓	✓				✓					✓	✓		✓			✓
Holstein, 2003[107]	✓	✓	✓	✓		✓		✓	✓			✓						✓	✓					✓
Holstein, 2003[109]	✓	✓	✓	✓		✓		✓	✓			✓							✓					
Holstein, 2009[102]	✓		✓	✓		✓		✓																
Holstein, 2011[103]	✓		✓	✓				✓																
Leese, 2003[25]	✓	✓	✓	✓				✓	✓		✓	✓						✓	✓		✓			✓
Miller, 2001[100]	✓	✓		✓			✓	✓			✓	✓						✓	✓		✓		✓	✓
Miller, 2010[89]	✓	✓		✓			✓				✓	✓											✓	✓
Quilliam, 2011[27]	✓	✓					✓											✓	✓	✓				✓
Sarkar, 2010[78]	✓		✓	✓		✓	✓	✓	✓			✓						✓	✓		✓			✓
Sato, 2010[106]	✓		✓	✓		✓	✓														✓			✓
Shen, 2008[101]						✓			✓															
Shorr, 1997[97]	✓	✓					✓				✓								✓		✓		✓	✓
Sotiropoulos, 2005[108]	✓	✓	✓								✓													
Stepka, 1993[98]											✓													
Sugarman, 1991[96]	✓	✓	✓															✓	✓				✓	
Whitmer, 2009[94]	✓	✓	✓						✓			✓	✓	✓				✓	✓		✓			✓
Zoungas, 2010[90]	✓	✓	✓	✓				✓	✓		✓	✓	✓			✓	✓	✓	✓		✓		✓	
TOTAL (31)																								

Table 6. Other Risk Factors in Multivariate Studies

Study, year	Other risk factors and multivariate controls
Akram, 2006[84]	*Risk Factors* Diabetes duration prior to insulin therapy (per 10 yrs) ↓, Treatment with ACE-I or ARB ↓ *Multivariate Controls* Hypertension, HTN therapy: RAS blocking, Non-RAS blocking, combination of both, Exercise, Use of tranquilizers
Bruce, 2009[92]	*Risk Factors* Inability to self manage medications ↑ *Multivariate Controls* "Clinically plausible variables"
Davis, 2010[16]	*Risk Factors* Lower FSG (less than or equal to 8.0 mmol/liter) ↑ *Multivariate Controls* English ability, Exercise in past 2 weeks, GAD antibody positive, Blood glucose self monitoring, Orthostatic hypotension, QTc interval (increase), Anticoagulant therapy, Regular ASA use, NSAID treatment, Allopurinol treatment, Fibrate therapy, Beta Blocker treatment, Hospitalized in 1998
Davis, 2011[93]	*Risk Factors* ACE-I use X, ACE DD genotype ↑ *Multivariate Controls* English ability, Exercise in past 2 weeks, GAD antibody positive, sulfonlyurea treatment, Blood glucose self monitoring, Anticoagulant therapy, Regular ASA use, NSAID treatment, Allopurinol treatment, Fibrate therapy, Beta Blocker treatment, Hospitalized in 1998 for hypoglycemia, Any hospitalization in past 12 months
Duran-Nah, 2008[104]	*Risk Factors* Attending physician (FP) ↑, Missed Meals ↑, Combined antihyperglycemic therapy ↑
Holstein, 2009[102]	*Risk Factors* KCNJ11 (E23K) gene X
Holstein, 2011[103]	*Risk Factors* Co-medication with other CYP2C9-main substrates ↑, CYP2C9-genotypes *2/*2, *2/*3, and *3/*3 X, Co-medication with other drugs being at least one CYP2C9-substrate X, Co-medication with angiotensin-converting enzyme inhibitor X, co-medication with analgesics X, Co-medication with gyrase inhibitors X, Presence of heart failure X, Previous participation at structured diabetes education X, Kind of accommodation (home vs nursing home) X *Multivariate Controls* Unspecified
Miller, 2001[100]	*Risk Factors* Follow-up fasting glucose X, Diabetes therapy increased at baseline visit X
Miller, 2010[89]	*Risk Factors* LDL level (> or equal to 2.59 mmol/l) ↓ *Multivariate Controls* Living arrangement (alone or with others), Systolic blood pressure, Use of beta blockers, Thiazolidinediones
Quilliam, 2011[27]	*Risk Factors* OADs: TZDs Continuous X, Intermittent X; Other OAD Continuous X, Intermittent X; Other medications: Allopurinol ↑, Benzodiazepine ↑, Beta-Blocker ↑, Blood glucose monitoring supplies ↓, Flouroquinolone ↑, NSAID ↑, Trimethoprim ↑; Charlson comorbidity (per 1 U change) ↑

**Predictors and Consequences of Severe Hypoglycemia
in Adults with Diabetes – Systematic Review of the Evidence**

Sarkar, 2010[78]	*Multivariate Controls* Non English language, Household Income, Self monitoring of blood glucose, Medication adherence
Shen, 2008[101]	*Multivariate Controls* Congestive heart failure, Depression, Hypertension, Health insurance status, Median income level
Shorr, 1997[97]	*Risk Factors* County of residence (rural vs. urban) X, Nursing home residence X, New hypoglycemia drug therapy ↑, Days since hospital discharge ↑ *Multivariate Controls* Duration of hypoglycemic drug use
Zoungas, 2010[90]	*Risk Factors* Two or more oral glucose lowering agents (yes vs. no) ↑

Table 7. Clinical Outcomes in Patients with Severe Hypoglycemia

Study, Year	All-Cause Mortality n/N (%)	MI, nonfatal n/N (%)	Stroke, non-fatal n/N (%)	Other Neurological Events (coma, seizures) n/N (%)
RANDOMIZED TRIALS				
Abraira, 1995[30] VA CSDM Group Standard Insulin (Std) vs. Intensive Tx (Int) N=153, men only, 40-69 yrs	NR	Int: 0% Std: 0%	NR	*Loss of consciousness* Int: 0/0 (0%) Std: 2/2 (100%) or 2/78 (2.6%) overall
ACCORD, 2008[3]; Bonds, 2011[61] Standard Tx (Std) vs. Intensive Tx (Int) N=10,251, 62% male, 40-79 yrs *p<0.05	*Definite role of hypoglycemia* Int: 1/816 (0.1%) Std: 0/256 (0%) *Probable role of hypoglycemia* Int: 1/816 (0.1%) Std: 2/256 (0.8%) *Possible role of hypoglycemia* Int: 25/816 (3.1%) Std: 13/256 (5.1%)	NR	NR	NR
ADVANCE, 2008;[4] Zoungas, 2010[90] Standard Tx (Std) vs. Intensive Tx (Int) N=11,140, 58% male, 55+ yrs	Int: 0/150 (0%) Std: 1/81 (1.2%) *Median follow-up of 5 years* ≥1 episode of severe hypoglycemia: 45/231 (19.5%) No severe hypoglycemia: 986/10,090 (9.0%) Adj HR=3.27 (95%CI 2.3-4.7)	NR	NR	NR
Arechavaleta, 2011[52] Sitagliptin vs. glimepiride (with metformin) N=1035, 54% male, mean age 56 yrs	Glimepiride: 0% Sitagliptin: 0%	NR	NR	Glimepiride: 6 episodes in 3 patients required medical assistance or were accompanied by neurological symptoms Sitagliptin: 1 episode in 1 patient
Buse, 2009[110] Lispro mix 75/25 vs. Glargine N=2091, 53% male, 30-80 yrs	NR	Lispro mix 75/25: 1/22 (4.5%) Glargine: 0/12 (0%)	NR	NR
Dailey, 2004[46] Glulisine vs. Regular human insulin N=876, 53% male, 18+ yrs	Glulisine: 0% Regular Human Insulin: 0%	NR	NR	NR
Duckworth (VADT), 2009[5] Standard Tx (Std) vs. Intensive Tx (Int) N=1791 Veterans, 97% male, mean age 60.4 yrs	NR	NR	NR	*Impaired consciousness* Int 9/100 pt year Std 3/100 pt year (p<0.001) *Complete loss of consciousness* Int 3/100 pt year Std 1/100 pt year; p<0.001
Heine, 2005[42] Exanatide vs. insulin glargine N=551; 56% male, 30-75 yrs *Reported that episodes of severe hypoglycemia resolved with oral carbohydrate and none required medical assistance or resulted in withdrawal from study	Exanatide: 0% Insulin glargine: 0%*	NR	NR	NR

Study, Year	All-Cause Mortality n/N (%)	MI, nonfatal n/N (%)	Stroke, non-fatal n/N (%)	Other Neurological Events (coma, seizures) n/N (%)
Holman, 2007,[111] Holman, 2009[43] Biphasic insulin aspart vs. prandial insulin aspart vs. basal insulin detemir N=708 (578 completed 3 yr follow-up), 64% male, 18+ yrs	No deaths related to hypoglycemia at 1 year follow-up (Holman, 2007)	NR	NR	*Loss of consciousness at 3-year follow-up (Holman, 2009)* Biphasic aspart: 1/235 (0.4%) Prandial asprt: 0/239 (0%) Basal detemir: 3/234 (1.3%)
Rašlová, 2004[112] Insulin detemir + insulin aspart vs. NPH + regular human insulin (HSI) N=395, 42% male, mean age 58 yrs	Insulin detemir + aspart: 0% NPH+ HIS: 0%	NR	NR	*Coma* Insulin detemir + aspart: 0% NPH+ HIS: 1/199 (0.5%)
Riddle, 2003;[41] Dailey, 2009[132] Bedtime glargine vs. NPH N=756, 56% male, 30-70 yrs	NR	NR	NR	Glargine: 0% NPH: 0%
Russell-Jones, 2009[54] Liraglutide, liraglutide placebo, or glargine N=576, 57% male, mean age 57 years	NR	NR	NR	Coma: 0% Seizures: 0%
UKPDS 33, 1998[21] Standard Tx (Std) vs. Intensive Tx (Int) N=3867, 61% male, 25-65 yrs	Int: 1/8 (12.5%) Std: 0/33 (0%)	NR	NR	NR
Williams-Herman, 2009 Sitagliptin vs. Metformin N=1091, 48% male, mean age 54 yrs	No deaths related to hypoglycemia	None	None	NR
COHORT STUDIES				
Davis, 2010[16] N=616, mean age 67 years, 52% male; mean follow-up of 6.4 years	0% (based on 66 episodes in 52 patients)	NR	NR	NR
Fadini, 2009[95] N=126, 44% male, mean age 77 yrs Patients admitted for hypoglycemia 2001-2007; 63 on oral meds, 63 on insulin	*In-hospital:* 2/126 (1.6%) due to irreversible hypoglycemia (treatment group not reported) *Total* deaths (at median follow-up of 23.2 months; cause of death not reported) On oral agent: 31.7% On insulin: 52.4%	NR	NR	Coma On oral agent: 54% On insulin: 30.2% (NOTE: the 2 deaths were due to irreversible hypoglycemia with seizures and shock)
Gürlek, 1999[116] N=114, 45% male, mean age 59 yrs Reviewed records of patients who frequently attended outpt clinic	No deaths among patients treated in a hospital setting	NR	NR	NR
Holstein, 2001[17] All emergency room patients with severe hypoglycemia Sulfonylurea-associated hypoglycemia only (all type 2) N=45, 36% male, mean age 83.5 yrs	0/45 (0%) at time of event 16/45 (35.6%) deaths during follow-up (mean of 22.8 months after event)	NR	NR	Coma: 23/45 (51%) Disorientation: 8/45 (18%) Somnolence: 5/45 (11%) Paralysis: 4/45 (9%) Cerebral seizures: 3/45 (7%) Psychological disturbances: 2/45 (5%)

Predictors and Consequences of Severe Hypoglycemia in Adults with Diabetes – Systematic Review of the Evidence

Study, Year	All-Cause Mortality n/N (%)	MI, nonfatal n/N (%)	Stroke, non-fatal n/N (%)	Other Neurological Events (coma, seizures) n/N (%)
Moen, 2009[75] N=243,222 Veterans (men and women) with at least 1 acute care hospitalization during 1 year study period and at least one glucose measurement (inpt or outpt) during study period	*Outpatient risk of death within one day of a hypoglycemic event (glucose <50 mg/dl)* OR=13.28 (9.30-19.18) for patients without chronic kidney disease (CKD) OR=6.84 (4.41-10.62) for patients with CKD (with glucose ≥ 70 mg/dl and no CKD as reference group)	NR	NR	NR
Shorr, 1997[97] N=586, 18% male, first episode of serious hypoglycemia, all age 65+, emergency room visit, hospitalization, or death	2/586 (0.3%)	3/586 (0.5%)	7/586 (1.2%)	Loss of consciousness: 49% of 598 episodes Seizures: 5% of 598 episodes Irrational behavior: 6% of 598 episodes TIA: 4/586 (0.7%)
Stepka, 1993[98] N=137, gender not reported, mean age 66 yrs Medical record data from patients hospitalized for "serious" hypoglycemia	Insulin: 7/101 (6.9%) Oral meds: 3/36 (8.3%)	NR	NR	NR
Sugarman, 1991[96] N=109 (126 admissions), 47% male, mean age 66 yrs Medical record data from hospitalizations associated with hypoglycemia in Navajo Indians with non-insulin-dependent diabetes	4/109 (3.7%) (only one death was attributed to hypoglycemia)	NR	NR	NR
OTHER STUDIES				
Asplund, 1991[105] N=19, 42% male, mean age 75 yrs, all taking glipizide Events reported to Swedish Adverse Drug Reactions Advisory Committee 1980-87	2/19 (11%) within 6 days of event Additional 1/19 (5.3%) within 23 days of event	NR	1/19 (5%) had stroke prior to hypoglycemic event with further functional impairment after event	*During event* Comatose: 11/19 (58%) Reduced conscious level: 3/19 (16%) *After event* Severe confusion: 2/19 (11%)
Ben-Ami, 1999[127] N=102, 40% male, median age 72 yrs, 90% type 2, admitted to a hospital with hypoglycemia(97%) or inpatient hypoglycemia (3%)	5/102 (5%)	Transient asymptomatic myocardial ischemia: 2/102 (2%)	NR	Seizure: 8/102 (8%) Transient right hemiplegia: 1/102 (1%)
Greco, 2010[128] N=99, 36% male, median age 84.7 yrs admitted for severe hypoglycemia (included only patients 80 or older)	0/99 (0%)	NR	NR	Coma: 19/99 (19%) Somnolence: 51/99 (51%) Reported cerebral seizures and/ or psychological disturbances in remaining patients
Hepburn, 1992[99] N=104, 50% male, mean age 63 yrs Interview with questionnaire about severe hypoglycemia in past year	NR	NR	NR	Convulsions: 3/86 (4%)

147

Study, Year	All-Cause Mortality n/N (%)	MI, nonfatal n/N (%)	Stroke, non-fatal n/N (%)	Other Neurological Events (coma, seizures) n/N (%)
Holstein, 2003[107] N=93 episodes, 41% male, mean age 78 yrs Physicians asked to report all episodes of severe sulfonylurea-associated hypoglycemia retrospectively or as they occurred NOTE: 6% of 400 contacted physicians responded	Glimepiride: 0/37 (0%) Glibenclaminde: 0/56 (0%)	NR	NR	*Severe brain damage* Glimepiride: 1/37 (2.7%) Glibenclaminde: (0%) *Presented with* Coma: 45% Disorientation: 18% Somnolence: 14% Cerebral seizure: 10% Local neuromuscular deficits: 8% Abnormal or inappropriate behavior: 5%
Holstein, 2003[109] Additional data from cohort described by Holstein, 2001 Insulin only (N=78) and insulin plus sulfonylurea (N=25) patients 41% male, mean age 76 yrs	0/148 (0%) in type 2 diabetic patients (1 death in non-diabetic patient with protracted spontaneous hypoglycemia)	NR	NR	NR
Sotiropoulos, 2005[108] Admitted to hospital due to severe hypoglycemia N=207, 41% male, mean age 62 yrs	0/207 (0%)	NR	2/207 (1.0%)	TIA: 2/207 (1.0%) *Presented with* Coma: 146/207 (71%) Semi-coma: 61/207 (29%) Convulsions: 3/207 (1.4%)
Stahl, 1999 N=28, 46% male, mean age 71.8 yrs Medical record data from patients admitted to emergency room for severe hypoglycemia	No hypoglycemia-related deaths (e.g., within 72 hrs of admission)	NR	NR	Coma or stupor at admission: 6/28 (21%)
Zargar, 2009[131] Patients with type 2 diabetes who were admitted to a medical center and who died with diabetes recorded on the death certificate N=693	Hypoglycemia was a cause of death in 22/693 (3.2%)	NR	NR	NR

Int = Intensive Treatment; Std = Standard Treatment; Tx = Treatment; NR = Not Reported; MI = Myocardial Infarction; TIA = Transient Ischemic Attack; CKD = Chronic Kidney Disease

Table 8. Other Outcomes in Patients with Severe Hypoglycemia

Study, Year	Hospitalizations n/N (%)	Emergency Department Visits n/N (%)	Accidents/ Trauma n/N (%)	Quality of Life	Other Outcomes	Type of Analysis 1=unadjusted; 2=minimal adjustment; 3=multivariate
RANDOMIZED TRIALS						
Abraira, 1995[30] VA-CSDM Group Std Insulin vs. Intensive Tx N=153, men only; 40-69 yrs	Intervention: 0% Control: 0%	NR	NR	NR	NR	NA
ADVANCE, 2008[4] Standard Tx (Std) vs. Intensive Tx (Int) N=11,140, 58% male, 55+ yrs	NR	NR	NR	NR	*Permanent disability* Int: 1/150 (0.7%) Std: 1/81 (1.2%)	NA
Arechavaleta, 2011[52] Sitagliptin vs. glimepiride N=1035, 54% male, mean age 56 yrs	NR	NR	NR	NR	Glimepiride: 6 episodes in 3 patients required medical assistance (location not specified) or were accompanied by neurological symptoms Sitagliptin: 1 episode in 1 patient	NA
Heine, 2005[42] Exanatide vs. insulin glargine N=551; 56% male, 30-75 yrs *Reported that episodes resolved with oral carbohydrate and none required medical assistance or resulted in withdrawal	Exanatide: 0% Insulin Glargine: 0%	Exanatide: 0% Insulin Glargine: 0%	NR	NR	NR	NA
Raslová, 2004[112] Insulin detemir + insulin aspart vs. NPH + regular human insulin (HSI) N=395, 42% male, mean age 58 yrs	Insulin detemir + aspart: 1/195 (0.5%) NPH + HSI: 2/199 (1.0%)	NR	NR	NR	NR	NA
Riddle, 2003;[41] Dailey, 2009[46] Bedtime glargine vs. NPH N=756, 56% male, 30-70 yrs	Glargine: 0% NPH: 0%	Glargine: 0% NPH: 2/13 events in 9 patients (15.4%)	NR	NR	*Withdrawal from study due to severe hypoglycemia* Glargine: 1/9 (12%) NPH: 3/9 (33%)	NA

Study, Year	Hospitalizations n/N (%)	Emergency Department Visits n/N (%)	Accidents/ Trauma n/N (%)	Quality of Life	Other Outcomes	Type of Analysis 1=unadjusted; 2=minimal adjustment; 3=multivariate
Russell-Jones, 2009[54] Liraglutide, liraglutide placebo, or glargine N=576, 57% male, mean age 57 years	NR	NR	NR	NR	*Medical Assistance* Liraglutide: 1/5 (20%) (no serious events in placebo or glargine groups)	NA
Williams-Herman, 2009[113] Sitagliptin vs. Metformin N=1091, 48% male, mean age 54 yrs	None	None	None	None	None	NA
COHORT STUDIES						
Bruce, 2009[92] N=205 with non-demented at initial assessment and who completed second assessment (83% of non-demented patients who were alive at 18 months) All ≥ 70 years	NR	NR	NR	NR	*Cognitive decline:* 33/205 (16%) (no difference in prior hypoglycemia episode between those with decline and those without) *Severe hypoglycemia:* more likely in patients with cognitive impairment (11.6%) or dementia (20.8%) than normal (3.0%) (p<0.01)	NA
Cobden, 2007[133] Patients converting from insulin syringe to biphasic pen device N=486 (subset of Lee, 2006)	Pre-pen: 8/44 hypoglycemic events (18%) Post-pen: 21/64 events (33%)	Pre-pen: 10/44 events (23%) Post-pen: 13/64 events (20%)	NR	NR	*Physician visits* Pre-pen: 15/44 events (34%) Post-pen: 21/64 events (33%) *Outpatient visits* Pre-pen: 4/44 events (9%) Post-pen: 6/64 events (9%)	NR
Fadini, 2009[95] N=126, 44% male, mean age 77 yrs Patients admitted for hypoglycemia 2001-2007; 63 on oral meds, 63 on insulin	All patients were hospitalized (study design)	Not applicable	*Falls* Oral meds: 25.4% Insulin: 17.5%	NR	*Acute coronary syndrome* Oral meds: 17.5% Insulin: 19.0% *Duration of hospital stay* Oral meds: 9.8 days Insulin: 8.0 days	NA
Goh, 2009[115] N=203 (192 or 95% Type 2), 37% male Patients admitted to observational ward in emergency department for hypoglycemia	22/203 (16%) transferred to inpatient team for longer period of treatment	All patients were seen in emergency department (study design)	NR	NR	151 patients were contacted at 7 and 28 days after discharge; 6/151 had recurrent hypoglycemia (2 were admitted)	NA

150

Study, Year	Hospitalizations n/N (%)	Emergency Department Visits n/N (%)	Accidents/ Trauma n/N (%)	Quality of Life	Other Outcomes	Type of Analysis 1=unadjusted; 2=minimal adjustment; 3=multivariate
Gürlek, 1999[116] N=114, 45% male, mean age 59 yrs Reviewed records of patients who frequently attended outpt clinic	0.05 episode/ patient/year	NR	NR	NR	NR	NA
Holstein, 2001[17] All emergency room patients with severe sulfonylurea-associated hypoglycemia (type 2) N=45, 36% male, mean age 83.5 yrs	All patients were hospitalized (study design)	14/45 (31%) initial treatment in emergency department	Soft tissue injuries or fractures: 6/45 (13%)	NR	NR	NA
Lee, 2006[114] Patients converting from insulin syringe to aspart pen (n=670) or biphasic pen (n=486) (see Cobden 2007 for subset data)	Pre-pen: 13/77 hypoglycemic events (17%) Post-pen: 41/139 events (30%) OR=0.88 (0.47-1.66)	Pre-pen: 12/77 events (16%) Post-pen: 19/139 events (14%) OR=0.44 (0.21-0.92)	NR	NR	*Physician visits* Pre-pen: 29/77 events (38%) Post-pen: 39/139 events (30%) OR=0.39 (0.24-0.64) *Outpatient visits* Pre-pen: 6/77 events (8%) Post-pen: 17/139 events (12%) OR=0.79 (0.31-2.01)	1
Leese. 2003[25] N=160 (57% type 2) with 244 hypoglycemic episodes, 54% male, mean age 52 years	52/244 episodes (21%)	19/244 episodes (8%) emergency or primary care visit 134/244 episodes (55%) ambulance + emergency or primary care visit	NR	NR	89/244 episodes (36%) ambulance service only	
Murata, 2005[19] Insulin-treated type 2 diabetes N=344 veterans, 96% male	2/55 severe episodes in 19 patients	NR	NR	NR	NR	NA
Nichols, 2010[26] Patients starting insulin N=2417, 49% male, mean age 60 yrs	No hospitalizations in 9970 patient-years of observation	NR	NR	NR	1.9% required medical contact for hypoglycemia in 1st year of insulin use; 0.4% by 5th year	NA

Predictors and Consequences of Severe Hypoglycemia in Adults with Diabetes – Systematic Review of the Evidence

Evidence-based Synthesis Program

Study, Year	Hospitalizations n/N (%)	Emergency Department Visits n/N (%)	Accidents/ Trauma n/N (%)	Quality of Life	Other Outcomes	Type of Analysis 1=unadjusted; 2=minimal adjustment; 3=multivariate
Panikar, 2003[117] Adding triple drug combination to insulin N=124, mean age 57 yrs, 47% male	2/28 (7.1%)	NR	NR	NR	NR	NA
Rhoads, 2005[118] N=2664, 69% male, mean age 45 yrs; insulin-treated type 1 and type 2	*Admissions per year* Hypoglycemia coding: 0.97 No hypoglycemia coding: 0.48 (p<0.01)	Visits per year Hypoglycemia coding: 0.85 No hypoglycemia coding: 0.40 (p<0.01)	NR	NR	*Short Term Disability Use* Hypoglycemia coding: 47% for mean of 19.5 days per P-Y No hypoglycemia coding: 32% for mean of 11.0 days per P-Y (both p<0.01)	NA
Shorr, 1997[97] N=586, first episode of serious hypoglycemia, all age 65+, emergency room visit, hospitalization, or death	Patients identified in hospital or emergency department	Patients identified in hospital or emergency department	Injury 10/586 (1.7%)	NR	NR	NA
Stepka, 1993[98] N=137, gender not reported, mean age 66 yrs Medical record data from patients hospitalized for "serious" hypoglycemia	NR	NR	*Bone injuries* Insulin: 10/101 (9.9%) Oral med: 0/36 (0%)	NR	NR	
Sugarman, 1991[96] N=109 (126 admissions), 47% male, mean age 66 yrs Medical record data from hospitalizations associated with hypoglycemia in Navajo Indians with non-insulin-dependent diabetes	4.7 per 1000 person-years	NR	NR	NR	NR	NA

Predictors and Consequences of Severe Hypoglycemia in Adults with Diabetes – Systematic Review of the Evidence

Study, Year	Hospitalizations n/N (%)	Emergency Department Visits n/N (%)	Accidents/ Trauma n/N (%)	Quality of Life	Other Outcomes	Type of Analysis 1=unadjusted; 2=minimal adjustment; 3=multivariate
Whitmer, 2009[94] N=16,667; 55% male, no prior diagnosis of dementia, mild cognitive impairment, or general symptom memory loss; mean follow-up of 3.8 years	NR	NR	NR	NR	*In patients who developed dementia:* History of at least one episode of severe hypoglycemia in prior 22 years: 17.0% No history of severe hypoglycemia: 10.3%	3 Positive graded association between severe hypoglycemia and risk of dementia; 2.39% increase in absolute risk of dementia per year in patients with h/o hypoglycemia compared to those without; adjusted Hazard Ratio for dementia : 1.44 (95% CI 1.25-1.66) for ≥ 1 episode vs. none
CROSS-SECTIONAL STUDIES						
Alvarez-Guisasola, 2010[119] Patients who added sulfonylurea or thiazolidinedione to metformin in past 5 years; age ≥ 30 yrs, 55% male	NR	NR	NR	*EQ-5D VAS by severity of hypoglycemic symptoms* None: 73.5 Mild: 71.0 Moderate: 65.8 Severe: 54.3 (p<0.0001) *Adjusted model* Severe symptoms associated with EQ-5D VAS (p<0.0001)	NR	3 age, gender, activity, weight, HbA1c, microvascular or cardiovascular history
Davis, 2005[120] N= 861; 58% male, 57% >65 yrs NOTE: response rate 30%	NR	NR	NR	*SF-36:* scores lower for patients with self-reported severe (vs. mild/moderate) hypoglycemia for all domains except vitality *EQ-5D:* lower scores for patients with severe (vs. mild/moderate)	*Productivity:* more days lost for severe (8.6) than mild/moderate (2.7); severity was predictor of productivity (p<0.05) *Resource use:* more contacts with health service for severe (13.2) than mild/moderate (11.5)	Adjusted for age, gender, diabetes complications, BMI, and type of diabetes

Predictors and Consequences of Severe Hypoglycemia
in Adults with Diabetes – Systematic Review of the Evidence

Study, Year	Hospitalizations n/N (%)	Emergency Department Visits n/N (%)	Accidents/ Trauma n/N (%)	Quality of Life	Other Outcomes	Type of Analysis 1=unadjusted; 2=minimal adjustment; 3=multivariate
Harsch, 2002[121] Surveys distributed at random in clinics, hospitals, education or self-help mtgs NOTE: data reported for oral anti-diabetic group (OA, 95% type 2, n=122, mean age 64 yrs) and conventional insulin group (CT, 72% type 2, n=151, mean age 59 yrs)	NR	NR	*Accidents per year driven on latest therapeutic regimen OA group: 2.05X10⁻³ CT group: 7.17X10⁻³ All type 2: 3.09X10⁻³ Hypoglycemia-induced accidents per year driven OA: 2/122 (1.6%) CT: 3/151 (2.0%) Symptomatic hypoglycemias per year driven (all Type 2): 0.04*	NR	*Breaks in driving caused by hypoglycemia OA group: 0.1 CT group: 0.2*	NA
Hermanns, 2005[122] N=388 (63% Type 2), 62% male, 35% age 18-48 yrs, 30% age 62+ yrs	NR	NR	NR	Severe hypoglycemia in past 12 months associated with increased risk for clinical (OR=4.4 [1.3-14.4]) and subclinical (OR=2.7 [1.1-6.9]) affective disorder but not anxiety disorder	*NR*	NA
Labad, 2010[123] Edinburgh Type 2 Diabetes Study N=1066, 51% male, mean age 68 yrs	NR	NR	NR	NR	Lifetime history of severe hypoglycemia (at least 1 episode) associated with symptoms of anxiety (ß=0.293, p<0.001) but not depression	Adjusted for gender, depression score, marital status, treatment for depression, diabetes treatment

154

**Predictors and Consequences of Severe Hypoglycemia
in Adults with Diabetes – Systematic Review of the Evidence**

Study, Year	Hospitalizations n/N (%)	Emergency Department Visits n/N (%)	Accidents/ Trauma n/N (%)	Quality of Life	Other Outcomes	Type of Analysis 1=unadjusted; 2=minimal adjustment; 3=multivariate
Leiter, 2005[124] N=133 with Type 2 DM, mean age 60 yrs 19 had severe episode in past 12 months; 34 reported episode in lifetime	See Emergency Department Visits	5.5% emergency or hospital visit	NR	*Lifestyle changes sometimes or always made after severe hypoglycemic episode (of n=19 reporting severe hypoglycemia in past 12 months)* Modified insulin dose: 58% Tested blood glucose more often: 84% Greater fear of future episode: 84% Additional concerns about driving: 16% Asked someone to check on them: 58% Went home from work, school, other activity: 32% Stayed home next day: 26%	*Additional physician visits:* 2.5% *Additional consultations:* 0.4% (unclear if denominator is 19 or 34 patients)	NA
Marrett, 2009;[81] Marrett, 2011[67] (additional analysis taking frequency into account) N=1984 (201 with severe or very severe hypoglycemic symptoms), 57% male, mean age 58 Data from 2007 National Health and Wellness Survey (NHWS)	NR	NR	NR	EQ-5D by severity (p<0.0001) Mild: 0.83 Moderate: 0.77 Severe/very severe: 0.67 HFS II worry by severity (p<0.0001) Mild: 12.3 Moderate: 20.1 Severe/very severe: 27.5 *Adjusted models:* Severe/very severe HFS II worry positively associated with and negatively associated with EQ-5D (both p<0.001) *EQ-5D decreased and HFS II worry increased as frequency of episodes increased*	NR	3 age, gender, BMI, education, duration of diabetes, HbA1c, diabetes complications

155

Study, Year	Hospitalizations n/N (%)	Emergency Department Visits n/N (%)	Accidents/ Trauma n/N (%)	Quality of Life	Other Outcomes	Type of Analysis 1=unadjusted; 2=minimal adjustment; 3=multivariate
Pettersson, 2011[82] Patients taking metformin and sulfonylurea for past 6 months (no insulin) N=430, 61% male, mean age 69 yrs	NR	NR	NR	*EQ-5D VAS score by severity* None: 0.76 Mild: 0.73 Moderate: 0.71 Severe: 0.68 Very severe: 0.66 (p=0.01 none/mild vs. moderate or worse) *EQ-5D dimensions with significant differences (none/ mild vs. moderate or worse)* Pain/discomfort: p=0.01 Anxiety/depression: 0=0.02 *HFS-II worry score by severity* None: 4 Mild: 7 Moderate: 8 Severe: 19 Very severe: 26 (p=0.06 none/mild vs. moderate or worse)		
Sarkar, 2010[78] N=14,357, 51% male, mean age 58 yrs	129/1579 (8%) hospital or ER OR=19.0 (13.0-26.0) compared to 1.6% of participants without significant hypoglycemia	see hospitalization	NR	NR	NR	

Study, Year	Hospitalizations n/N (%)	Emergency Department Visits n/N (%)	Accidents/ Trauma n/N (%)	Quality of Life	Other Outcomes	Type of Analysis 1=unadjusted; 2=minimal adjustment; 3=multivariate
Vexiau, 2008[126] Patients taking sulfonylurea and metformin for at least 6 months N=400, 54% male, mean age 62 yrs	NR	NR	NR	EQ-5D summary score by symptom severity (p=0.04) None: 0.80 Mild: 0.73 Moderate: 0.70 Severe/very severe: 0.54 Worry score by symptom severity (p=0.02) None: 10.2 Mild: 16.5 Moderate: 22.2 Severe/very severe: 25.3 Severe hypoglycemia significantly associated with HFS-II worry and EQ-5D summary scores (p<0.0001)	NR	3 Adjusted for age, gender, marital status, education, activity, duration of DM, history of microvascular events, major medical events, adequate glycemic control
OTHER STUDIES						
Asplund, 1991[105] N=19, 42% male, mean age 75 yrs, all taking glipizide Events reported to Swedish Adverse Drug Reactions Advisory Committee 1980-87	NR	NR	NR	NR	*Prolonged hypoglycemia (23-60 hours):* 5/19 (26%)	
Ben-Ami, 1999[127] N=102, 40% male, median age 72 yrs, 90% type 2, admitted to a hospital with hypoglycemia (97%) or inpatient hypoglycemia (3%)	All patients were hospitalized (study design)	Not applicable	7/102 (7%)	NR	Protracted hypoglycemia (12-72 hours): 40/102 (39%)	
Greco, 2010[128] admitted for severe hypoglycemia N=99, 36% male, median age 84.7 yrs	Median hospitalization 5.5 days (cohort defined by hospitalization)	NR	NR	NR	Protracted hypoglycemia (12-72 hrs): 61/99 (61%)	

Predictors and Consequences of Severe Hypoglycemia in Adults with Diabetes – Systematic Review of the Evidence

Study, Year	Hospitalizations n/N (%)	Emergency Department Visits n/N (%)	Accidents/ Trauma n/N (%)	Quality of Life	Other Outcomes	Type of Analysis 1=unadjusted; 2=minimal adjustment; 3=multivariate
Hemmelgarn, 2006[135] All drivers 67 to 84 years old NOTE: mix of type 1 and type 2 *RR=Rate Ratio; reference is no anti-diabetic therapy in preceding year ^Sulfonylurea + Metformin; no increased risk with oral monotherapy	NR	NR	*Injurious motor vehicle crash* Any insulin: RR*=1.3 (95% CI 1.0-1.8) Insulin only: RR=1.4 (95% CI 1.0-2.0) Combined oral^: RR=1.3 (95% CI 1.0-1.7) with dose response	NR	NR	Adjusted for age, gender, previous motor vehicle crashes, place of residence
Hepburn, 1992[99] N=104, 50% male, mean age 63 yrs Interview with questionnaire about severe hypoglycemia in past year	NR	NR	*Injury (not defined)*: 4/86 (5%)	NR	NR	
Holstein, 2003[107] N=93 episodes, 41% male, mean age 78 yrs Physicians asked to report all episodes of severe sulfonylurea-associated hypoglycemia retrospectively or as they occurred	NR	NR	NR	NR	*Prolonged severe hypoglycemia (>12 hr)* Glimepiride: 8/37 (22%) Glibenclamide: 5/56 (9%)	
Lundkvist, 2005[125] N=309, 60% male, mean age 65 yrs	0/7 (0%)	3 visits among 6 pts requiring healthcare for hypoglycemia in past month	NR	NR	8 nurse visits, 3 physician visits, 1 telephone contact with medical care among 6 patients requiring healthcare for hypoglycemia in past month	

Predictors and Consequences of Severe Hypoglycemia in Adults with Diabetes – Systematic Review of the Evidence

Study, Year	Hospitalizations n/N (%)	Emergency Department Visits n/N (%)	Accidents/ Trauma n/N (%)	Quality of Life	Other Outcomes	Type of Analysis 1=unadjusted; 2=minimal adjustment; 3=multivariate
Redelmeier, 2009[129] N=795, 84% male, mean age 52 yrs; reported to vehicle licensing authorities for review	NR	NR	*Severe hypoglycemia in past 2 years 34/57 (60%) who had crash 200/738 (27%) without crash OR=4.07 (2.35-7.04)*	NR	NR	1
Stahl, 1999[28] N=28, mean age 71.8 yrs Medical record data from patients admitted to emergency room for severe hypoglycemia	All patients were hospitalized (study design)	NR	NR	NR	*Prolonged hypoglycemia: 1/28 (3.6%)*	1
Stork, 2007[130] Driver's license for ≥ 2 yrs; at least 8000 km driven in past year N=20 type 2, 80% male, mean age 52 yrs Induced hypoglycemia (2.7 mmol/l)	NR	NR	NR	NR	*11/20 (55%) felt hypoglycemic:* 5/11 (45%) would measure glucose 6/11 (55%) would not drive 9/20 (45%) "maybe" felt hypoglycemic: 3/9 (33%) would drive 2/9 (22%) "maybe" drive 2/9 (22%) would measure glucose 2/9 (22%) would not drive	

NR = Not reported; N/A = Not Applicable

159

APPENDIX F. FOREST PLOTS FOR KEY QUESTION #1

Appendix F, Figure 1.

Severe hypoglycemia event rates for insulin glargine studies*

Group By Duration	Study Name	Event Rate	Lower Limit	Upper Limit	Total
long-term	Rosenstock 2009	0.074	0.054	0.100	38 / 513
long-term	Buse 2011	0.029	0.016	0.050	12 / 419
long-term	Rosenstock 2008	0.027	0.014	0.054	8 / 291
long-term		0.041	0.019	0.084	58 / 1223
short-term	Kennedy 2006	0.030	0.026	0.034	228 / 7607
short-term	Riddle 2003	0.025	0.013	0.046	9 / 367
short-term	Heine 2005	0.015	0.006	0.039	4 / 267
short-term	Davies 2005	0.010	0.008	0.013	45 / 4588
short-term	Rosenstock 2001	0.004	0.001	0.027	1 / 259
short-term		0.016	0.008	0.032	288 / 13088
Overall		0.025	0.015	0.041	346 / 14311

Event rate and 95% CI: −0.25, −0.13, 0.00, 0.13, 0.25

*Alone or added to OHAs

Appendix F, Figure 2.

Severe hypoglycemia event rates for insulin detemir studies

Group By Duration	Study Name	Event Rate	Lower Limit	Upper Limit	Total
long-term	Holman 4T 2009	0.009	0.002	0.034	2 / 234
long-term	Rosenstock 2008	0.017	0.007	0.041	5 / 291
long-term		0.014	0.007	0.029	7 / 525
moderate-term	Marre 2009	0.004	0.001	0.009	4 / 1129
moderate-term		0.004	0.001	0.009	4 / 1129
Overall		0.009	0.005	0.015	11 / 1154

Event rate and 95% CI: −0.25, −0.13, 0.00, 0.13, 0.25

Appendix F, Figure 3.

Severe hypoglycemia event rates for NPH insulin studies

Group By Duration	Study Name	Event Rate	Lower Limit	Upper Limit	Total
long-term	Rosenstock 2009	0.109	0.085	0.139	55 / 504
long-term		0.109	0.085	0.139	55 / 504
short-term	Rosenstock 2001	0.023	0.010	0.051	6 / 259
short-term		0.023	0.010	0.051	6 / 259
Overall		0.093	0.073	0.118	61 / 763

Event rate and 95% CI: −0.25, −0.13, 0.00, 0.13, 0.25

Appendix F, Figure 4.

Severe hypoglycemia event rates for NPH insulin studies*

Group By Duration	Study Name	Event Rate	Lower Limit	Upper Limit	Total
long-term	Rosenstock 2009	0.109	0.085	0.139	55 / 504
long-term		0.109	0.085	0.139	55 / 504
short-term	Frische 2003	0.026	0.012	0.056	6 / 232
short-term	Rosenstock 2001	0.023	0.010	0.051	6 / 259
short-term	Riddle 2003	0.018	0.009	0.037	7 / 389
short-term	Rayman (glulisine) 2007	0.004	0.001	0.018	2 / 448
short-term	Dailey (glulisine) 2004	0.014	0.006	0.030	6 / 435
short-term	Rayman (RHI) 2007	0.016	0.008	0.033	7 / 442
short-term	Dailey (RHI) 2004	0.011	0.005	0.027	5 / 441
short-term		0.016	0.012	0.022	39 / 2646
Overall		0.050	0.041	0.061	94 / 3150

Statistics for Each Study — Event rate and 95% CI

Scale: -0.25   -0.13   0.00   0.13   0.25

*NPH insulin as either primary therapy or in combination (Frische, sulfonylurea; Riddle oral OHAs; Rayman and Dailey, glulisine or regular insulin)

Appendix F, Figure 5.

Severe hypoglycemia events, NPH insulin versus insulin glargine studies*

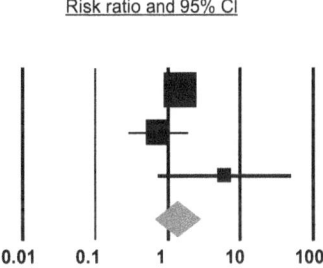

Study Name	Risk Ratio	Lower limit	Upper limit	NPH insulin	Insuline glargine
Rosenstock 2009	1.473	0.993	2.186	55 / 504	38 / 513
Riddle 2003	0.734	0.276	1.950	7 / 389	9 / 367
Rosenstock 2001	6.000	0.727	49.489	6 / 259	1 / 259
	1.367	0.666	2.806	68 / 1152	48 / 1139

Events / Total — Risk ratio and 95% CI

Scale: 0.01   0.1   1   10   100

Appendix F, Figure 6.

Severe hypoglycemia event rates for insulin lispro studies

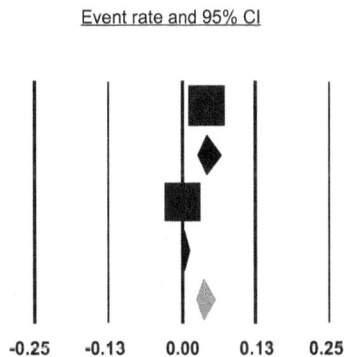

Group By Duration	Study Name	Event Rate	Lower Limit	Upper Limit	Total
long-term	Buse 2011	0.042	0.027	0.064	20 / 476
long-term		0.042	0.027	0.064	20 / 476
short-term	Anderson 1997	0.001	0.000	0.010	1 / 722
short-term		0.001	0.000	0.010	1 / 722
Overall		0.036	0.023	0.054	21 / 1198

Statistics for Each Study — Event rate and 95% CI

Scale: -0.25   -0.13   0.00   0.13   0.25

Appendix F, Figure 7.

Severe hypoglycemia event rates for insulin aspart studies

Group By Duration	Study Name	Event Rate	Lower Limit	Upper Limit	Total	Event rate and 95% CI
long-term	Holman 4T 2009 (Prandial)	0.021	0.009	0.049	5 / 239	
long-term	Holman 4T 2009 (Biphasic)	0.026	0.012	0.056	6 / 235	
long-term		0.023	0.013	0.042	11 / 474	
short-term	Bentrop 2011 (Biphasic)	0.002	0.000	0.007	2 / 1154	
short-term	Liebl 2009 (Biphasic)	0.003	0.000	0.043	0 / 178	
short-term	Valensi IMPROVE 2009 (Biphasic)	0.001	0.001	0.002	69 / 52419	
short-term		0.001	0.002	0.002	71 / 53751	
Overall		0.002	0.002	0.002	82 / 54225	

*Subjects may also have received OHAs in addition to insulin aspart.

-0.25   -0.13   0.00   0.13   0.25

Appendix F, Figure 8.

Severe hypoglycemia event rates for insulin glulisine (+NPH insulin) short-term (26 wks) studies

Study Name	Event Rate	Lower limit	Upper limit	Total	Event rate and 95% CI
Rayman 2006	0.004	0.001	0.018	2 / 448	
Daily 2004	0.014	0.006	0.030	6 / 435	
	0.009	0.003	0.026	8 / 883	

-0.25   -0.13   0.00   0.13   0.25

Appendix F, Figure 9.

Severe hypoglycemia rates for sulfonylurea studies*

Group By Duration	Study Name	Event Rate	Lower Limit	Upper Limit	Total	Event rate and 95% CI
long-term	Holstein 2001	0.013	0.009	0.017	44 / 3489	
long-term		0.013	0.009	0.017	44 / 3489	
moderate-term	Matthews 2011	0.010	0.006	0.016	15 / 1546	
moderate-term	Seck 2010	0.015	0.008	0.029	9 / 584	
moderate-term	Garber 2011	0.002	0.000	0.031	0 / 248	
moderate-term	Marre 2009	0.004	0.000	0.066	0 / 114	
moderate-term		0.011	0.007	0.017	24 / 2492	
short-term	UK Hypoglycemia Group	0.074	0.037	0.141	8 / 108	
short-term	Arechavaleta 2011	0.015	0.008	0.031	8 / 519	
short-term	Nauck 2009	0.002	0.000	0.032	0 / 242	
short-term	Russell-Jones 2009	0.004	0.000	0.066	0 / 114	
short-term	Chou 2008	0.002	0.000	0.034	0 / 225	
short-term	Kendall 2005	0.002	0.000	0.031	0 / 247	
short-term	Drouin 2004	0.001	0.000	0.009	1 / 800	
short-term	Schernthaner 2004	0.001	0.000	0.009	0 / 845	
short-term		0.005	0.001	0.019	17 / 3100	
Overall		0.012	0.009	0.015	85 / 9081	

*Sulfonylurea monotherapy and combined sulfonylurea and metformin studies

-0.25   -0.13   0.00   0.13   0.25

Appendix F, Figure 10.

Severe hypoglycemia events for BARI 2D study, insulin sensitization versus insulin provision

Study name	Risk ratio	Lower limit	Upper limit	Events/Total Sensitization	Provision
BARI 2D 2009	0.642	0.479	0.861	68 / 1153	106 / 1154
	0.642	0.479	0.861	68 / 1153	106 / 1154

Risk ratio and 95% CI

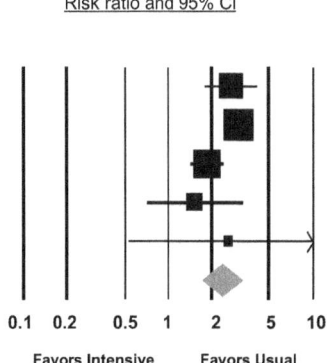

0.1   0.2   0.5   1   2   5   10

Favors Sens.   Favors Prov.

Appendix F, Figure 11.

Severe hypoglycemia events for intensive glycemic control versus usual care studies

Study name	Risk ratio	Lower limit	Upper limit	Events/Total Intensive control	Usual care
VADT 2009	2.736	1.792	4.177	76 / 892	28 / 899
ACCORD 2008	3.096	2.717	3.527	849 / 5128	274 / 5123
ADVANCE 2008	1.884	1.442	2.463	150 / 5571	81 / 5669
UKPDS-33 1998	1.529	0.708	3.299	33 / 3071	8 / 1138
VA-CSDM 1995	2.600	0.520	12.993	5 / 75	2 / 78
	2.396	1.757	3.268	1113 / 14737	393 / 12907

Risk ratio and 95% CI

0.1   0.2   0.5   1   2   5   10

Favors Intensive   Favors Usual